THE SUPER EASY & PRACTICAL MEDITERRANEAN DIET COOKBOOK FOR BEGINNERS

─── ★★★ ───

Optimize Your Health with Budget Friendly,
Quick & Tasty, 30-Minute, 5-Ingredient, Heathy Recipes

ELENA FLORENZ

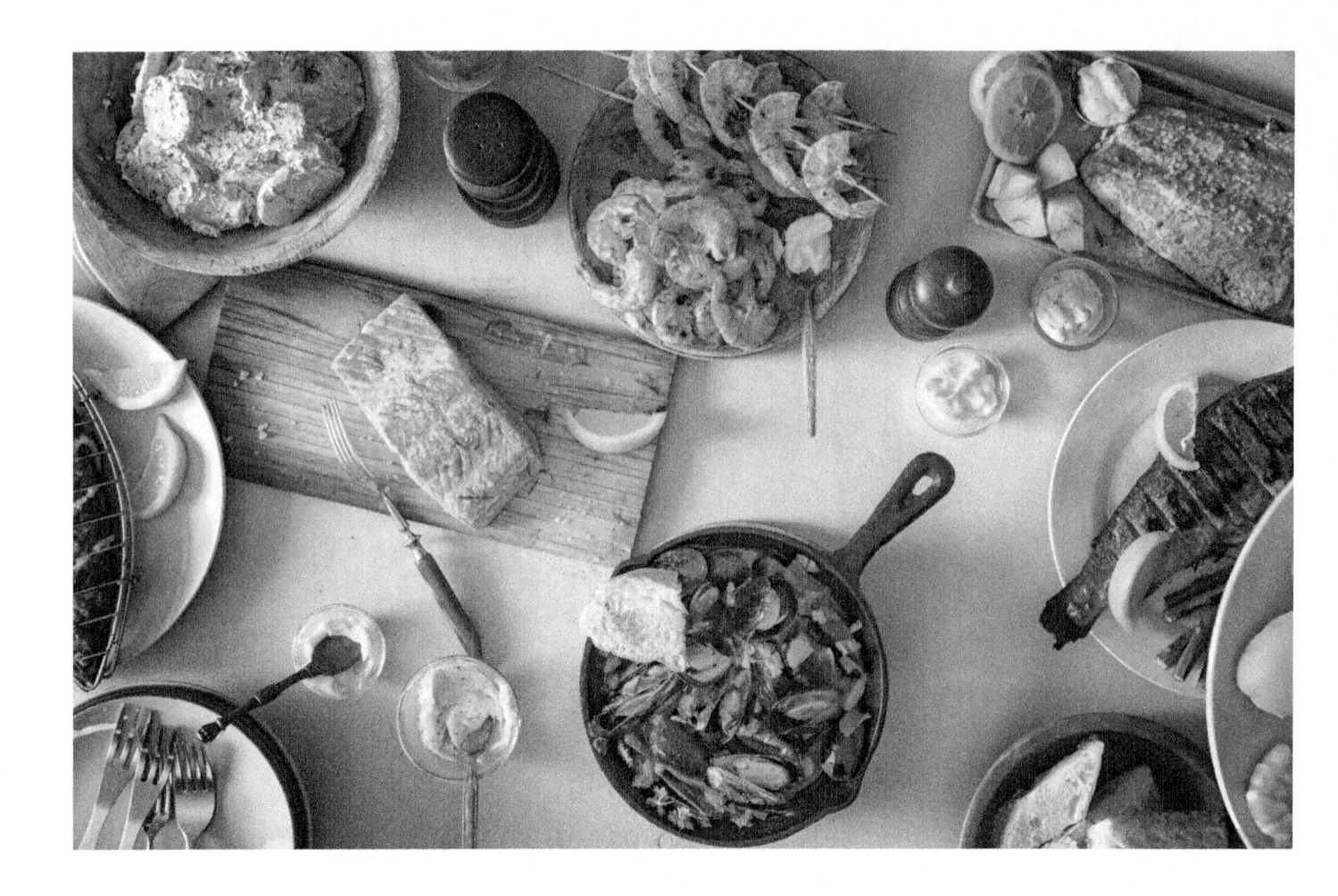

COPYRIGHT © 2024 BEGINNERS

All rights reserved. No part of this book may be reproduced, distributed, or transmitted in any form or by any means, including photocopying, recording, or other electronic or mechanical methods, without the prior written permission of the publisher, except in the case of brief quotations embodied in critical reviews and certain other noncommercial uses permitted by copyright law.

LEGAL NOTICE. The information contained in this book is intended for educational and informational purposes only and is not a substitute for professional medical advice or treatment. Consult with a qualified healthcare professional before making any changes to your diet or lifestyle. The author and publisher expressly disclaim responsibility for any adverse effects that may result from the use or application of the information contained in this book.

DISCLAIMER. While every effort has been made to ensure the accuracy and reliability of the information contained in this book, neither the author nor the publisher can assume responsibility for errors, inaccuracies, or omissions. The reader is advised to consult with healthcare providers for specific health-related issues and should exercise caution when preparing recipes, particularly for allergies and dietary restrictions.

CONTENTS

YOUR JOURNEY TO HEALTHIER, HAPPIER LIVING — 7

CHAPTER 1
INTRODUCTION TO THE MEDITERRANEAN DIET — 8

DOWNLOAD YOUR BONUS
SUPER EASY MEDITERRANEAN RECIPE BOOK WITH VIBRANT, FULL COLOR PICTURES — 12

CHAPTER 2
DIPS, SAUCES AND CONDIMENTS — 13

Creamy Tahini-Lemon Dip — 14
Roasted Red Pepper Hummus — 14
Zesty Garlic Herb Dip — 14
Sun-Dried Tomato Pesto — 14
Lemon-Caper Vinaigrette — 14
Lemon-Herb Yogurt Dip — 15
Garlic-Lemon Aioli — 15
Smoky Paprika Yogurt Dip — 15
Cucumber-Mint Raita — 15
Classic Tzatziki — 15
Spicy Harissa Dip — 15
Olive Tapenade — 16
Creamy Feta Dip — 16
Garlic-Infused Olive Oil Drizzle — 16

CHAPTER 3
BREAKFASTS — 17

Savory Tomato-Basil Omelet — 18
Sweet Almond and Fig Barley with Vanilla and Coconut — 18
Greek Yogurt with Honey, Walnuts, and Spiced Raisin Syrup — 18
Mediterranean Scramble with Lemon Zest and Spinach — 18
Lemon Herb Millet Porridge Garlic-Infused Oil — 19
Frittata — 19
Orange and Pistachio Breakfast Bowl with Almond Flakes and Mint — 19
Spiced Sweet Potato & Date Delight — 19
Homemade Labneh — 20
Simple Caprese Medley — 20
Mediterranean Avocado and Nut Bowl with Lemon-Oregano Drizzle — 20
Zaatar and Olive-Infused Gluten Free Pita — 21
Sunrise Quinoa Delight — 21
Parsley Olive Tapenade on Rice Cakes — 21
Cardamom-Spiced Barley and Caramelized Pear Medley — 21
Mediterranean Stuffed Avocado Boats with Tomato, Olive & Herb Filling — 22
Lemon Zucchini Quinoa Bowl with Herb-Infused Olive Oil — 22
Garlic-Infused Tomato-Basil Crostini with Balsamic Glaze — 22
Mediterranean-Spiced Tofu Scramble with Bell Peppers and Tomato — 23
Bourekas — 23
Pistachio Chia Banana Bowl — 23
Cinnamon Figs & Seeds Porridge — 23
Manakish with Feta and Ground Meat — 24
Pomegranate & Walnut Greek Yogurt Parfait — 24
Smoky Sweet Potato Breakfast Hash — 24
Sun-Kissed Chickpea and Avocado Breakfast Bowl — 24
Stuffed Sweet Potato with Avocado, Pomegranate & Toasted Seeds — 25
Apple-Almond Delight Breakfast Bowl — 25
Sun-Dried Tomato Chickpea Pancakes with Herbed Toppings — 25
Tropical Avocado Mango Bowl — 25

CHAPTER 4
APPETIZERS, MEZE, TAPAS, SMALL PLATES — 26

Spiced Mini Peppers with Hummus and Herbs — 27
Crispy Za'atar Chickpeas with Garlic — 27
Basil-Infused Tomato Crostini — 27
Zesty Cucumber Feta Bites — 27
Spinach & Pine Nut Puff Rolls — 28
Balsamic Marinated Mushrooms with Fresh Herbs — 28
Herbed Labneh Balls with Lemon & Pistachios — 28
Stuffed Grape Leaves with Quinoa & Veggies — 28
Paprika Deviled Egg — 29
Warm Feta with Honey and Thyme — 29
Grilled Eggplant with Pine Nuts — 29
Spinach and Feta Phyllo Triangles — 29
Cucumber and Mint Gazpacho Shots — 30
Sun-Dried Tomato and Olive Tapenade — 30
Marinated Artichokes and Olives Medley — 30
Spinach & Chickpea Bruschetta — 30

Roasted Cauliflower and Chickpea Bowl — 31
Lentil and Veggie Lettuce Wraps — 31
Fresh Cucumber & Tomato Avocado Toast — 31
Cucumber and Feta Rolls with Lemon Zest — 32
Stuffed Mushrooms with Sun-Dried Tomato and Feta — 32
Crispy Sweet Potato and Chickpea Patties — 32

CHAPTER 5
SOUPS — 33

Creamy Broccoli and Leek Soup — 34
Zucchini & Basil Bliss Soup — 34
Spicy Beetroot and Ginger Delight Soup — 34
Creamy Potato Leek Soup — 34
Smoky Chicken and Butternut Squash Soup — 35
Turmeric Lemon Chickpea Soup — 35
Velvety Parsnip and Apple Soup — 35
Cod and Potato Chowder — 36
Herb Beef Soup — 36
Creamy Pea and Sweet Potato Soup — 36
Roasted Butternut Squash and Cauliflower Soup — 36
Lemon Chicken and Vegetable Orzo Soup — 37
Spicy Shrimp and Fennel Citrus Soup — 37
Hearty Turkey Meatball and Kale Soup — 37
Spinach-Chickpea Comfort Soup — 37
Zucchini-Infused Chicken Soup — 38
Ocean Kissed Tomato Soup with Sea Bass — 38
Spiced Lamb and Vegetable Soup — 38
Minestrone Soup — 38
Creamy Salmon Soup — 39

YOUR FREE BONUSES! — 39

CHAPTER 6
SALADS — 40

Simple Greek Salad with Lemon-Olive Dressing — 41
Grilled Zucchini and Tomato Salad with Lemon Herb Dressing — 41
Zesty Quinoa Power Salad — 41
Grilled Chicken with Mixed Greens in Creamy Herb Dressing — 41
Lemon Kissed Grilled Chicken Salad — 42
Grilled Steak Salad with Balsamic Vinaigrette — 42
Fattoush Salad — 42
Grilled Chicken and Roasted Bell Pepper Salad with Tahini-Garlic Dressing — 42
Garden Fresh Watermelon-Cucumber Salad — 43
Tuna and White Bean Salad with Creamy Mustard Dressing — 43
Roasted Carrot And Arugula Salad with Dijon Vinaigrette — 43
Mediterranean-Inspired Lentil Parsley Salad — 43
Grilled Mediterranean Salmon Salad with Avocado Dressing — 44
Roasted Cauliflower and Chickpea Salad with Lemon-Tahini Dressing — 44
Vibrant Veggie Chickpea Salad — 44
Tabbouleh — 44
Shrimp and Cucumber Citrus Salad — 45
Crunchy Rainbow Salad with Honey-Lime Dressing — 45
Spicy Avocado & Quinoa Corn Salad — 45
Shrimp and Mango Medley with Cilantro Dressing — 46
Turkey and Pear Salad with Honey Mustard Dressing — 46
Chickpea and Arugula Salad with Tahini Dressing — 46

CHAPTER 7
VEGETABLES — 47

Roasted Zucchini, Squash and Cherry Tomatoes with Red Onion — 48
Green Bean Medley with Roasted Garlic and Almond Bliss — 48
Baked Stuffed Zucchini Boats with Spinach and Bell Pepper — 48
Mediterranean Roasted Asparagus Medley — 48
Rosemary-Parsnip Bake with Almond Crust — 49
Savory Caramelized Onion & Mushroom Medley — 49
Stir-Fried Snap Peas with Sesame and Mushrooms — 49
Cinnamon-Spiced Roasted Carrots with Sweet Potato, Parsnips and Chili — 50
Spaghetti Squash with Spinach and Pine Nuts — 50
Roasted Kohlrabi with Almond Crumble — 50
Grilled Artichokes with Rosemary — 51
Braised Fennel with Pistachios — 51
Stuffed Acorn Squash with Quinoa & Tomatoes — 51
Spaghetti Squash with Tomato and Basil Sauce — 52
Roasted Bell Peppers with Olive Tapenade — 52
Steamed Artichokes with Avocado Tahini Dressing — 52
Miso Glazed Bok Choy — 53
Grilled Portobello Mushrooms on Spinach Bed with Balsamic Glaze — 53
Sautéed Celeriac with Shallots — 53
Swiss Chard Rolls Stuffed with Lentil Rice — 53
Sautéed Kale with Lemon and Garlic — 54

Grilled Eggplant and Roasted Pepper Stew – 54
Creamy Cauliflower and Leek Mash – 54
Spiced Cauliflower Rice with Peas, Carrots, and Cilantro – 54
Zucchini Noodles with Almond Pesto and Roasted Vegetables – 55
Stuffed Veggie Portobello Mushrooms – 55
Braised Turnips with Miso and Scallions – 55
Cauliflower and Spinach Stir-Fry with Almond – 56
Roasted Brussels Sprouts with Lemon and Garlic – 56
Steamed Broccolini with Sesame Dressing – 56
Stuffed Tomatoes with Lentils and Herbs – 56
Roasted Vegetables with Honey Lemon Glaze – 57
Coconut Turmeric Vegetable Stew – 57
Caramelized Rutabaga with Miso Glaze – 57
Braised Leeks with Almonds and Chickpeas – 58
Braised Fennel with White Beans and Tomatoes – 58
Leeks with Mustard Cream Sauce – 58
Fennel and Radish Slaw – 58
Grilled Delicata Squash with Hazelnuts and Orange Zest – 59
Celery Root Steaks with Capers and Dill – 59
Artichoke Hearts with Spinach-Almond Filling – 59

CHAPTER 8
WHOLEGRAINS, BEANS AND PASTA – 60

Crispy Persian Rice – 61
Egyptian Fava Beans – 61

Mediterranean Bowl with Quinoa, Hummus, and Harissa – 61
Cranberry Apple Freekeh Stuffing – 61
Greek Lemon Rice – 62
Black Bean Avocado Quinoa Bowl – 62
Beans and Greens over Polenta – 62
Green Beans and Potatoes – 62
Lebanese Green Beans with Olive Oil – 63
Rigatoni with Creamy Ricotta and Spinach – 63
Lentils and Rice with Caramelized Onions – 63
Risotto Radicchio and Gorgonzola – 63
Pasta with Chickpeas – 64
Tunisian Chickpea Stew – 64
Greek Baked Beans – 64
Freekeh – 64
Garbanzo Bean Pilaf – 65
Balilah – 65
Risotto alla Puttanesca – 65
Black Olive Tapenade With Pasta – 65
Buckwheat Pancakes – 66
White Beans with Tahini – 66
Turkish Lentil Mezze – 66
Tuna Pasta with Peas – 66
Sicilian Almond Pasta – 67
Spanish Rice and Beans – 67
Creamy Orzo with Garlic, Parmesan and Blistered Tomatoes – 67
Butter Beans with Garlic, Lemon & Herbs – 67
Toasted Orzo with Parmesan and Sundried Tomatoes – 68
Lebanese Rice with Vermicelli – 68
Farro Risotto – 68
Garlic Parmesan White Beans – 68

CHAPTER 9
FISH & SEAFOOD – 69

Mussels with Chorizo – 70
Grilled Oysters – 70

Spicy Couscous Recipe with Shrimp – 70
Spanish Seafood Pasta – 70
Tuna Rillettes – 71
Moroccan Fish Kofta – 71
Linguine with Clams – 71
Spaghetti with Garlicky Sautéed Shrimp – 72
Egyptian Fried Fish Sandwich – 72
Tunisian Salad – 72
Mussels Marinara with Fennel (Greece) – 72
Greek Fish with Onions and Tomatoes – 73
Seafood Paella – 73
Mediterranean Salmon Kabobs – 73
Cod with Tomato Sauce – 74
Shrimp Fra Diavolo – 74
Lemony Shrimp Risotto – 74
Fish en Papillote, Mediterranean-style – 74
Za'atar Garlic Salmon – 75
Lemon Garlic Shrimp with Peas and Artichokes – 75
Mediterranean Lemon Poached Halibut – 75
Mediterranean Oven Roasted Spanish Mackerel – 76
Mediterranean-Style Whole Roasted Red Snapper – 76
Steamed Mussels in Garlic White Wine Broth – 76
Stuffed Tomatoes with Tuna – 76
Mediterranean Fish Fillet – 77
Grilled Cod, Gyro-Style – 77
Easy Mediterranean Sautéed Scallops – 78
Turkish-Style Marinated Salmon – 78
Greek Salmon – 78
Persian Stuffed Fish – 78

CHAPTER 10
POULTRY AND MEAT – 79

Baked Chicken Thighs – 80
Roast Turkey Breast – 80
Baked Tomato Chicken Thighs with Couscous – 80
Greek Meatballs and Potatoes – 81
Sheet Pan Za'atar Chicken with Veggies – 81
Pastilla (Skillet Chicken Pie) – 81
Roast Chicken with Citrus and Honey – 82
Italian Steak with Arugula and Parmesan – 82
Sun-Dried Tomato Chicken – 82
Pan Seared Lamb Chops – 82
Chicken Saltimbocca – 83
Stifado (Greek Beef Stew) – 83
Greek Chicken Marinade – 83
Greek Meatloaf Wrapped in Grape Leaves – 84
Chicken in Tomato Sauce – 84
Garlic Dijon Chicken – 84
Kleftiko (Greek Lamb Cooked in Parchment) – 84
Moroccan Meatballs – 85
Sausage and Lentils with Fennel – 85
Moussaka – 85
Joojeh Kabob – 86
Shish Kabob – 86
Baked Boneless Chicken Thighs with Baharat – 86
Skillet Mushroom Chicken – 86
Greek Lamb Stew with Orzo – 87
Italian Meatballs in Tomato Sauce – 87
Moroccan-Inspired Chicken Couscous – 87
Apricot Chicken – 88
Chicken Tagine – 88
Albondigas (Spanish Meatballs) – 88

CHAPTER 11
EGGS – 89

White Bean Shakshuka – 90
Spanakopita Egg Muffins – 90
Italina Eggs in Purgatory – 90
Halloumi Cheese with Egg – 90
Dijon Deviled Eggs – 91
Turkish Poached Eggs – 91
Eggs Fra Diavolo – 91
Tuna Deviled Eggs – 91
Lebanese Potatoes and Eggs – 91
Tunisian Brik au Thon – 92
Turkish Spinach and Eggs – 92
Soft Scrambled Eggs with Chives – 92
Za'atar Olive Oil Fried Eggs – 92
Oven Baked Eggs – 92

CHAPTER 12
BAKED GOODS – BREADS, FLATBREADS, PIZZAS, WRAPS – 93

Pita Breakfast Pizza – 94
Vegetarian Pizza – 94
Mediterranean Wrap – 94
Majorcan Vegetable Flatbread – 94
Palestinian Flatbread – 95
Chicken Gyro – 95
Eggplant Pizza – 95
Turkish Steak Wraps – 96
Greek New Year's Bread – 96
Flatbread – 96
Sesame Bread Rings – 97
Greek Pizza – 97
Phyllo-Wrapped Greek Baked Feta with Honey – 97
Persian Flatbread – 97

CHAPTER 13
DESSERTS – 98

French Pear Tart – 99
Pignoli Cookies – 99
Mango Strawberry Smoothie with Greek Yogurt – 99
Pear Cake – 99
Traditional Greek Orange Cake – 100
Chocolate Hazelnut Cookies – 100
Lemon Sorbet – 100
Poached Apricots with Ricotta – 100
Candied Almonds – 101
Tiramisu – 101
Fruit Salad with Citrus Honey Dressing – 101
Greek Rice Pudding – 101
Rose Water Milk Pudding – 102
Italian Carrot Cake – 102
Burbura – 102
Crema Catalana – 102
Berry Compote – 103
Italian Chocolate Cake – 103
Tahini Banana Date Shake – 103
Fig Pastry – 103

MEAL PLAN 1-7 DAYS – 104

MEAL PLAN 8-14 DAYS – 105

MEAL PLAN 15-22 DAY – 106

MEAL PLAN 23-30 DAY – 107

CONVERSIONS AND EQUIVALENTS – 108

CONCLUSION – 109

THANK YOU – 110

REFERENCES – 111

YOUR JOURNEY TO HEALTHIER, HAPPIER LIVING

Hi there, and welcome! If you're holding this book, chances are you're ready to make some positive changes to your life. Whether your goal is to feel better, eat healthier, or simplify your cooking routine, I want you to know—you're in the right place.

The Mediterranean diet has been called the "healthiest diet on the planet," and for good reason. But let's be honest—changing the way you eat can feel overwhelming, especially when life is already so busy. That's exactly why I created *The Super Easy & Practical Mediterranean Diet Cookbook for Beginners: Optimize Your Health with Budget Friendly, Quick & Tasty, 30-Minute, 5-ingredient Healthy Recipes + A 30-Day Meal Plan*. This book is all about making it as simple (and delicious) as possible for you to adopt this incredible lifestyle.

Here's what you'll find inside:

- **A high volume of recipes with 290 quick and easy recipes**. The collection of recipes will give you a *diverse variety* of flavors, textures, and cooking techniques—no matter how much time or experience you have.
- **30-minute meals** using just 5 ingredients (excluding pantry staples like oil, salt, and herbs) that are *healthy yet packed with flavor and budget friendly*— perfect for busy days when time is tight.
- A **30-day meal plan** with shopping lists to make planning and prepping a breeze.
- **Two bonus ebooks**:
  - **Meal Prep and Food Repurposing Guide** where you'll find *practical tips* for saving money, repurposing ingredients, and minimizing food waste.
  - **A Reference Book of 70 Classic Mediterranean Recipes with Full Colored Pictures** - an extract of classic and more complex dishes where vibrant, full-colored photos will form the foundational compass to make more dishes with confidence.

It may feel daunting initially as you embark on this journey. Maybe you're worried about giving up your favorite meals. Or maybe you think it's too expensive or time-consuming. Fret not, this cookbook is here to show you how to *ease* into the Mediterranean diet and help you incorporate small changes into your everyday life that add up to big results.

The truth is, the Mediterranean diet isn't just about food. It's a way of life that's centered on balance, joy, and connection. From wholesome ingredients to the beauty of shared meals, this lifestyle has been proven to support better heart health, reduce the risk of chronic illnesses, and even improve your mood.

It's about a celebration of life, rather than a diet. And I'll be here with you every step of the way, sharing recipes, tips, and tools to make this transition as smooth and enjoyable as possible.

Let's get started—one delicious bite at a time.

To your health and happiness,
Elena Florenz

CHAPTER 1

INTRODUCTION TO THE MEDITERRANEAN DIET

"Good food is the foundation of genuine happiness and lasting health."

A JOURNEY INTO HEALTH AND FLAVOR

The Mediterranean diet is more than a way of eating—it's a lifestyle that celebrates health, joy, and connection. Rooted in centuries-old traditions, this approach has nourished some of the world's healthiest and happiest communities. By adopting it, you're embracing a way of life that balances delicious meals with overall well-being.

The Mediterranean diet isn't about restrictions or complexity—it's about savoring wholesome ingredients, fostering connections, and finding joy in every meal. With this book, you'll not only nourish your body but also embrace a lifestyle that supports physical, emotional, and mental well-being.

Your journey to health and flavor begins here. Let's make it as enjoyable—and delicious—as possible.

THE TIMELESS ORIGINS OF THE MEDITERRANEAN DIET

The Mediterranean diet is more than just a modern health trend—it's a way of life with roots stretching back thousands of years.

Emerging from the sun-soaked regions of Greece, Italy, and Spain, it was shaped by the local environment and culture. Ancient communities thrived on fresh, local ingredients like olives, grains, fruits, vegetables, nuts, seeds, and fish, while meat was consumed sparingly.

Olive oil, revered as "liquid gold" since 5000 BCE, became a cornerstone, symbolizing health and prosperity.

This diet reflected a lifestyle of balance, sustainability, and harmony with nature, where meals were opportunities to gather, relax, and nourish both body and soul.

Embracing the Mediterranean Lifestyle: Food, Family, and Well-Being

The Mediterranean diet is more than just a way of eating—it's a celebration of balance, joy, and connection. Imagine sitting around a sun-drenched table with loved ones, sharing vibrant meals and laughter. For the Mediterranean, this is everyday life.

Food isn't just fuel; it's a way to build community. Meals bring people together, creating bonds that reduce loneliness and spark joy. The secret to Mediterranean happiness lies in balancing good food, good company, and a mindful approach to living.

This lifestyle teaches us to:

- **Savor the Simple Things**: Fresh produce, ripe tomatoes, outdoor dining experience.
- **Connect Through Food**: Sharing meals turns ordinary moments into celebrations.
- **Embrace Balance**: Enjoying food and life in a natural, joyful way.

The Mediterranean way isn't just about eating—it's a tradition of health, vitality, and well-being. So set the table, invite loved ones, and enjoy the simple joys of life, one delicious bite at a time.

The Power of Shared Meals: Nourishing Body and Soul

In the Mediterranean lifestyle, shared meals offer more than just nourishment—they foster connection, community, and well-being. Whether it's a casual weekday meal or a festive gathering, eating together provides numerous physical and emotional benefits:

- **Reduces Stress and Boosts Mood**: Eating together fosters conversation and laughter, which lowers stress and enhances emotional well-being.

- **Strengthens Bonds**: Shared meals create quality time, deepen relationships, and build lasting memories.

- **Encourages Healthier Habits**: Eating together promotes mindful eating, helping to slow down, enjoy food, and make healthier choices.

- **Better Nutrition and Lower Obesity Risk**: Families who eat together consume more fruits and vegetables, and home-cooked meals provide healthier portions, reducing the risk of obesity.

- **Improved Mental Health**: Regular shared meals help reduce anxiety, depression, and stress, while fostering emotional closeness and connection.

The Science Behind the Health Benefits of the Mediterranean Diet

The Mediterranean diet isn't about restriction; it's about balance and nourishing your body with wholesome, nutrient-rich foods. Here's how it supports overall health:

- **Heart Health**: Healthy fats from olive oil and omega-3s in fish help reduce bad cholesterol (LDL) and boost good cholesterol (HDL), lowering the risk of heart disease.

- **Reduced Inflammation**: Antioxidants in fruits, vegetables, and nuts fight inflammation, which is linked to chronic diseases like cancer and arthritis.

- **Weight Management**: Fiber-rich foods such as whole grains and legumes stabilize blood sugar and keep you full longer, promoting healthy weight loss.

- **Cognitive Health**: Antioxidants and healthy fats protect brain cells, reducing the risk of cognitive decline and diseases like Alzheimer's.

- **Lean Proteins**: Focus on lean meats like fish and poultry, which provide protein without the harmful saturated fats found in red meat.

- **Natural Anti-Inflammatories**: Herbs like oregano, turmeric, and nuts help reduce chronic inflammation, which is a root cause of many diseases.

Incorporating these healthy fats, fiber, lean proteins, and antioxidants into your diet can reduce the risk of heart disease, diabetes, cognitive decline, and inflammation-related diseases, while promoting overall well-being and longevity.

Principles of the Mediterranean Diet

The Mediterranean Diet is simple, flavorful, and filled with wholesome ingredients. These guiding principles help bring out the best health benefits:

- **Focus on Plant-Based Foods**: Fruits, vegetables, whole grains, legumes, nuts, and seeds make up the bulk of the diet.

- **Healthy Fats Are Key**: Instead of butter or margarine, olive oil is the go-to fat, providing heart-healthy benefits.

- **Moderate Protein from Seafood**: Fish, especially fatty types like salmon and sardines, are consumed regularly.

- **Limited Red Meat and Sweets**: Red meats and sugary treats are eaten only occasionally.

- **Enjoy with Friends and Family**: The Mediterranean way isn't just about food—it's about sharing meals with loved ones, savoring every bite, and making dining a joyful experience.

- **Regular Physical Activity**: Walking, gardening, and other forms of light exercise are essential to the Mediterranean lifestyle.

FOODS TO EAT AND AVOID

What to Eat

1. **Fruits and Vegetables**:
   Aim for a rainbow of colors—think tomatoes, leafy greens, bell peppers, berries, and citrus fruits. They're packed with vitamins, antioxidants, and fiber to support overall health.

2. **Whole Grains**:
   Choose whole-grain bread, brown rice, oats, and barley for sustained energy and improved digestion.

3. **Healthy Fats**:
   Use extra virgin olive oil as your go-to fat. Include avocados, nuts (like almonds and walnuts), and seeds for heart health and inflammation reduction.

4. **Fish and Seafood**:
   Enjoy salmon, tuna, mackerel, and shellfish a few times a week for brain-boosting omega-3s and lean protein.

5. **Legumes**:
   Lentils, chickpeas, and beans provide plant-based protein and fiber, keeping you full and your blood sugar steady.

6. **Herbs and Spices**:
   Flavor dishes with fresh herbs like basil, oregano, rosemary, and garlic to reduce the need for salt and benefit from their anti-inflammatory properties.

7. **Dairy in Moderation**:
   Opt for low-fat Greek yogurt and small amounts of cheese like feta and Parmesan.

What to Avoid

1. **Processed Foods**:
   Skip ultra-processed snacks, fast foods, and ready-made meals high in additives.

2. **Refined Grains**:
   Avoid white bread, refined pasta, and pastries, which lack fiber and nutrients.

3. **Sugary Drinks**:
   Limit soft drinks, energy drinks, and excessive fruit juices.

4. **Red and Processed Meats**:
   Reduce intake of bacon, sausages, and steaks.

5. **Added Sugars**:
   Steer clear of sweets, candies, and sugary cereals.

Key Ingredients and Their Benefits

- **Olive Oil**:
  Known as "liquid gold," olive oil is rich in antioxidants and monounsaturated fats, reducing inflammation and supporting heart health, skin, and hormonal balance.

- **Fruits and Vegetables**:
  Full of vitamins, minerals, and antioxidants that boost immunity, promote glowing skin, and support eye health.

- **Herbs and Spices**:
  Basil, oregano, rosemary, and thyme not only enhance flavor but also reduce inflammation and support overall health.

- **Fish and Seafood**:
  Rich in omega-3 fatty acids, they protect your brain, heart, and joints.

- **Legumes and Whole Grains**:
  High in fiber and protein, these staples help with digestion, keep you full, and stabilize blood sugar.

TIPS FOR TRANSITIONING TO THE MEDITERRANEAN DIET

Switching to a new way of eating can feel overwhelming, but it doesn't have to be. Here are some simple tips to help you transition seamlessly:

- **Start Small**: Incorporate a Mediterranean dish into one meal a day, such as a salad with olive oil or a whole-grain side dish.

- **Stock Your Pantry**: Keep staples like olive oil, canned beans, and whole grains on hand for quick and easy meals.

- **Plan Ahead**: Use the meal plan provided in this book to save time and stay consistent.

- **Experiment with Flavors**: Try new herbs, spices, and ingredients to keep your meals exciting and flavorful.

HOW TO USE THIS BOOK

Embarking on a healthier lifestyle with the Mediterranean diet can feel like a big step, but this book is designed to make it easy and enjoyable. Here's a quick guide to get the most out of it:

1. **Start with the Basics**
   Discover the history, principles, and science of the Mediterranean diet to understand why it's so effective. If you're pressed for time, skim the "Principles" section for a quick rundown of what to eat and avoid.

2. **Follow the 30-Day Meal Plan**
   Ease into the diet with a 30-day meal plan, complete with shopping lists. It's a simple roadmap that takes the stress out of meal prep, offering a variety of delicious meals.

3. **Explore Quick and Easy Recipes**
   Browse the heart of the book—quick, simple, budget-friendly recipes categorized by meal type. Find dishes ready in 30 minutes or less using just five main ingredients.

4. **Dive Into the Bonuses**
   Check out tips on meal prep, bulk cooking, and reducing food waste. These sections will save you time and money while keeping your kitchen efficient.

5. **Personalize Your Journey**
   Adapt the recipes to your taste. Make this diet your own—skip seafood, go heavy on fresh herbs, or add your unique twist.

6. **Embrace the Lifestyle**
   The Mediterranean diet is more than food—it's about enjoying meals with loved ones, staying active, and savoring each bite. Use the lifestyle tips to enrich your daily routine.

7. **Refer to the Key Ingredients Guide**
   Build a Mediterranean pantry with the essential ingredient guide. Keep it handy for grocery shopping and meal planning.

8. **Take It One Step at a Time**
   Start small—swap one meal, add more veggies, or use olive oil instead of butter. Progress, not perfection, is the goal.

This book is your guide to a flavorful, healthy Mediterranean lifestyle. You've got all the tools you need—let's begin creating meals that nourish your body, mind, and soul!

DOWNLOAD YOUR BONUS
SUPER EASY MEDITERRANEAN RECIPE BOOK WITH VIBRANT, FULL COLOR PICTURES

A Reference Book of 70 Classic Mediterranean Recipes with Full Colored Pictures

A collection of signature dishes comes alive with vibrant, full-colored photos forming a foundational compass so you can identify the key elements that make up a dish in a food group.

Making you more confident in creating delectable Mediterranean dishes.

Get access to this vibrant recipe booklet and other bonus ebooks by copying the below link and pasting it in your browser or scanning the QR code with your mobile phone's camera.

https://heartbookspress.com/SuperEasyMediterranean-FreeBonuses

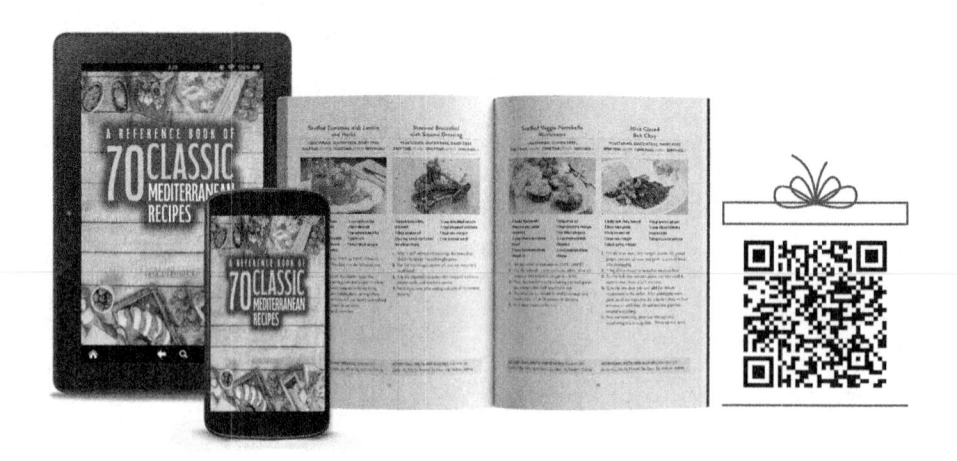

CHAPTER 2

DIPS, SAUCES AND CONDIMENTS

From the sun-drenched coasts of Greece to the vibrant markets of Morocco, the Mediterranean region is a treasure trove of culinary delights. Explore a collection of dips, sauces, and condiments that capture the essence of this diverse and flavorful cuisine.

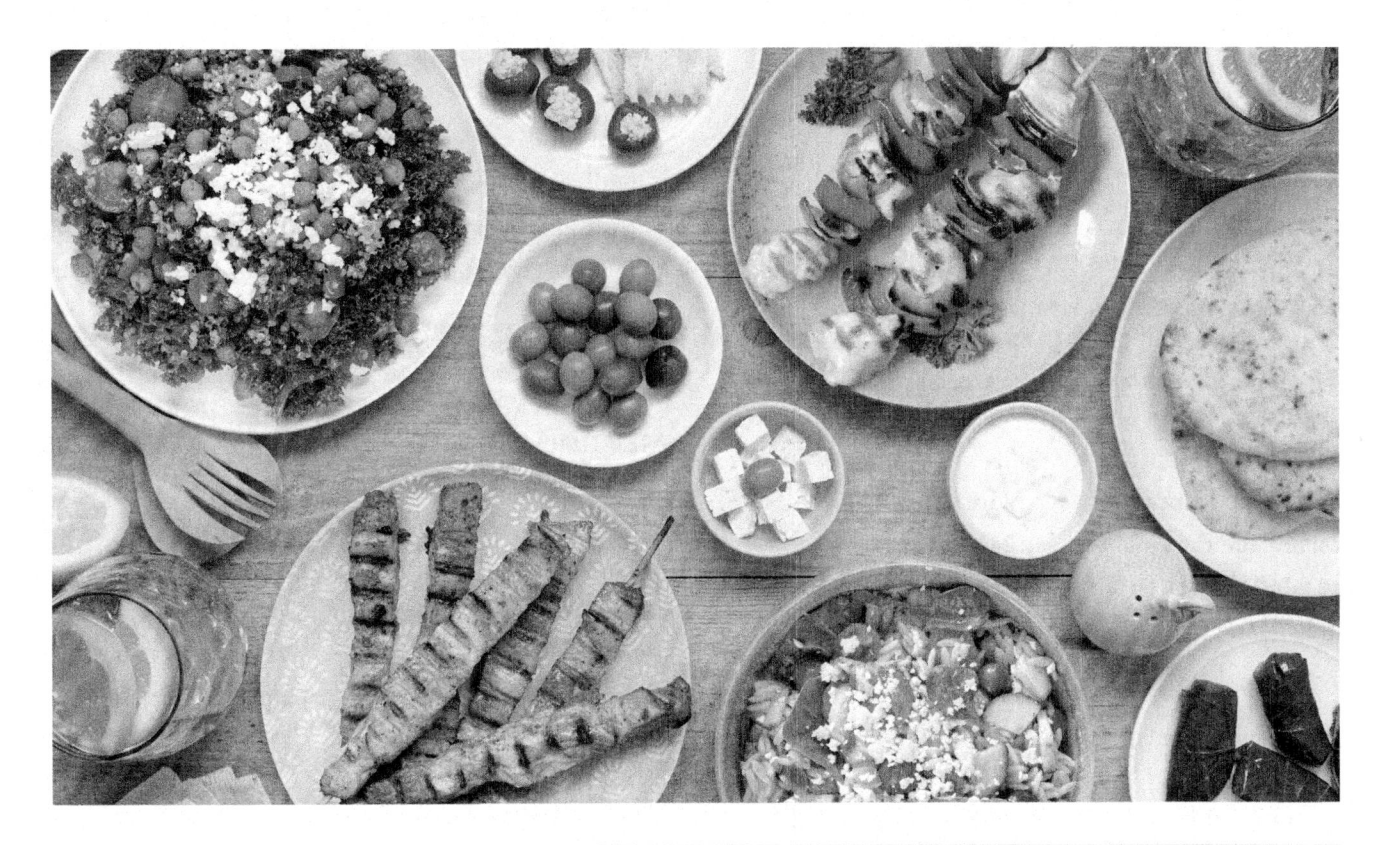

TIPS

- Store your dips and sauces in airtight containers in the refrigerator. For longer storage, consider freezing.

- Use fresh herbs, toasted nuts, or crumbled cheese to garnish your dips and sauces.

- Pair your dips and sauces with homemade breads, crackers, or pita chips for a complete appetizer experience.

Creamy Tahini-Lemon Dip

VEGETARIAN, GLUTEN FREE, DAIRY FREE
PREP TIME: 05 MIN **COOK TIME:** 00 MIN **SERVINGS:** 4
Calories: 70, Carbs: 2g, Fat: 6g, Protein: 2g, Fiber: 1g, Sodium: 290mg

- 3 tbsp tahini
- 2 tbsp freshly squeezed lemon juice
- 1 clove garlic, minced
- 2-3 tbsp water (as needed for consistency)
- ½ tsp salt

1. Whisk the lemon juice and tahini together in a small bowl.
2. Add salt and minced garlic. Stir thoroughly.
3. One tablespoon at a time, gradually whisk in water until the dip reaches the consistency you want.
4. If needed, taste and adjust the salt.

Roasted Red Pepper Hummus

VEGETARIAN, GLUTEN FREE, DAIRY FREE
PREP TIME: 10 MIN **COOK TIME:** 00 MIN **SERVINGS:** 6
Calories: 90, Carbs: 6g, Fat: 6g, Protein: 3g, Fiber: 2g, Sodium: 85mg

- 1 cup canned chickpeas, drained and rinsed
- 1 roasted red bell pepper, peeled and chopped
- 2 tbsp tahini
- 2 tbsp olive oil
- 1 clove garlic, minced

1. In a food processor or blender, combine the chickpeas, roasted red bell pepper, tahini, olive oil, and garlic.
2. Blend until it's smooth. If necessary, add a little water to change the consistency.
3. If desired, add salt after tasting.

Zesty Garlic Herb Dip

VEGETARIAN, GLUTEN FREE
PREP TIME: 05 MIN **COOK TIME:** 00 MIN **SERVINGS:** 4
Calories: 30, Carbs: 2g, Fat: 0g, Protein: 3g, Fiber: 0g, Sodium: 190mg

- ½ cup plain Greek yogurt
- 1 tbsp freshly squeezed lemon juice
- 1 clove garlic, minced
- 1 tbsp fresh dill, chopped
- ½ tsp salt

1. Combine Greek yogurt and lemon juice in a small bowl.
2. Add the salt, dill, and garlic and stir until thoroughly blended.
3. To improve flavor, chill for five minutes before serving.

Sun-Dried Tomato Pesto

VEGETARIAN, GLUTEN FREE, DAIRY FREE
PREP TIME: 10 MIN **COOK TIME:** 00 MIN **SERVINGS:** 6
Calories: 80, Carbs: 3g, Fat: 7g, Protein: 1g, Fiber: 1g, Sodium: 110mg

- ½ cup sun-dried tomatoes (packed in oil, drained)
- 2 tbsp olive oil
- 1 clove garlic, minced
- 2 tbsp pine nuts
- ¼ tsp salt

1. In a food processor, combine sun-dried tomatoes, garlic, and olive oil.
2. Add salt and pine nuts. Smoothly pulse.
3. If necessary, adjust the oil and salt for consistency.

Lemon-Caper Vinaigrette

VEGETARIAN, GLUTEN FREE, DAIRY FREE
PREP TIME: 05 MIN **COOK TIME:** 00 MIN **SERVINGS:** 4
Calories: 90, Carbs: 0g, Fat: 10g, Protein: 0g, Fiber: 0g, Sodium: 45mg

- 3 tbsp olive oil
- 1 tbsp freshly squeezed lemon juice
- 1 tsp capers, finely chopped
- ½ tsp Dijon mustard
- 1 pinch black pepper

1. Whisk the lemon juice and olive oil together in a small bowl.
2. Add black pepper, Dijon mustard, and capers and stir until emulsified.
3. Pour over roasted veggies or salads.

Lemon-Herb Yogurt Dip

VEGETARIAN, GLUTEN FREE
PREP TIME: 05 MIN **COOK TIME:** 00 MIN **SERVINGS:** 4
Calories: 25, Carbs: 1g, Fat: 0g, Protein: 2g, Fiber: 0g, Sodium: 70mg

- ½ cup plain Greek yogurt
- 1 tbsp freshly squeezed lemon juice
- 1 pinch salt
- 1 tsp fresh parsley, finely chopped
- 1 tsp fresh dill, finely chopped

1. Whisk the lemon juice and Greek yogurt together in a bowl until smooth.
2. Add salt, dill, and parsley and stir. Stir thoroughly.
3. For optimal flavor, chill for five minutes prior to serving.

Garlic-Lemon Aioli

GLUTEN FREE, DAIRY FREE
PREP TIME: 05 MIN **COOK TIME:** 00 MIN **SERVINGS:** 4
Calories: 95, Carbs: 1g, Fat: 10g, Protein: 0g, Fiber: 0g, Sodium: 120mg

- ½ cup mayonnaise
- 1 tbsp freshly squeezed lemon juice
- 1 clove garlic, minced
- 1 tsp olive oil
- 1 pinch salt

1. Whisk the lemon juice and mayonnaise together in a small bowl.
2. Add salt, garlic, and olive oil. Mix until it's smooth.
3. Use as a sandwich spread or dipping sauce.

Smoky Paprika Yogurt Dip

VEGETARIAN, GLUTEN FREE
PREP TIME: 05 MIN **COOK TIME:** 00 MIN **SERVINGS:** 4
Calories: 30, Carbs: 2g, Fat: 2g, Protein: 2g, Fiber: 0g, Sodium: 200mg

- ½ cup plain Greek yogurt
- 1 tsp smoked paprika
- 1 tbsp olive oil
- ½ tsp garlic powder
- ¼ tsp salt

1. In a bowl, mix together Greek yogurt and smoked paprika.
2. Add salt, garlic powder, and olive oil and stir. Stir thoroughly.
3. Before serving, let it cool for five minutes.

Cucumber-Mint Raita

VEGETARIAN, GLUTEN FREE
PREP TIME: 10 MIN **COOK TIME:** 00 MIN **SERVINGS:** 4
Calories: 25, Carbs: 2g, Fat: 1g, Protein: 2g, Fiber: 0g, Sodium: 60mg

- ½ cup plain Greek yogurt
- ¼ cup grated cucumber (squeeze out excess water)
- 1 tbsp fresh mint, chopped
- 1 pinch cumin powder
- 1 pinch salt

1. In a bowl, combine grated cucumber and Greek yogurt.
2. Add the salt, cumin powder, and mint and stir until combined.
3. Serve cold as a side dish or with pita.

Classic Tzatziki

VEGETARIAN, GLUTEN FREE
PREP TIME: 10 MIN **COOK TIME:** 00 MIN **SERVINGS:** 6
Calories: 35, Carbs: 2g, Fat: 2g, Protein: 3g, Fiber: 0g, Sodium: 60mg

- ½ cup plain Greek yogurt
- ¼ cup grated cucumber (squeezed dry)
- 1 clove garlic, minced
- 1 tbsp olive oil
- 1 tbsp lemon juice

1. In a bowl, combine Greek yogurt and cucumber.
2. Add lemon juice, olive oil, and garlic and stir. Mix thoroughly.
3. Serve cold as a spread or dip.

Spicy Harissa Dip

VEGETARIAN, GLUTEN FREE, DAIRY FREE
PREP TIME: 05 MIN **COOK TIME:** 00 MIN **SERVINGS:** 4
Calories: 45, Carbs: 3g, Fat: 3g, Protein: 1g, Fiber: 1g, Sodium: 120mg

- 2 tbsp harissa paste
- ½ cup plain dairy-free yogurt
- 1 tbsp olive oil
- 1 pinch smoked paprika
- ¼ tsp salt

1. Mix the dairy-free yogurt and harissa paste in a small bowl until smooth. Add salt, smoked paprika, and olive oil and stir.
2. If desired, add extra harissa to increase the amount of spiciness.

Olive Tapenade

VEGETARIAN, GLUTEN FREE, DAIRY FREE
PREP TIME: 10 MIN **COOK TIME:** 00 MIN **SERVINGS:** 4
Calories: 95, Carbs: 1g, Fat: 10g, Protein: 0g, Fiber: 1g, Sodium: 290mg

- **1 cup pitted black olives**
- **1 tbsp capers**
- **1 clove garlic, minced**
- **2 tbsp olive oil**
- **1 tbsp lemon juice**

1. In a food processor, coarsely grind the garlic, capers, and olives.
2. Pour in lemon juice and olive oil. Pulse until well blended.
3. Use as a spread or as a topping.

Creamy Feta Dip

VEGETARIAN, GLUTEN FREE
PREP TIME: 10 MIN **COOK TIME:** 00 MIN **SERVINGS:** 6
Calories: 80, Carbs: 2g, Fat: 6g, Protein: 4g, Fiber: 0g, Sodium: 260mg

- **½ cup crumbled feta cheese**
- **¼ cup plain Greek yogurt**
- **1 tbsp olive oil**
- **1 tsp dried oregano**
- **1 pinch black pepper**

1. Use a fork to mash the feta cheese in a bowl.
2. Add the olive oil and Greek yogurt and stir until smooth.
3. Add black pepper and oregano. Mix to blend.

Garlic-Infused Olive Oil Drizzle

GLUTEN FREE, DAIRY FREE
PREP TIME: 10 MIN **COOK TIME:** 00 MIN **SERVINGS:** 6
Calories: 80, Carbs: 0g, Fat: 9g, Protein: 0g, Fiber: 0g, Sodium: 10mg

- **½ cup extra virgin olive oil**
- **2 cloves garlic, thinly sliced**
- **1 pinch chili flakes**
- **½ tsp dried oregano**
- **1 pinch salt**

1. In a small saucepan, heat the olive oil over low heat.
2. Add the chili flakes and pieces of garlic. Cook the garlic gently for about 5 minutes, or until it is aromatic and golden.
3. Take off the heat and mix in the salt and oregano.
4. Before spreading it over salads, roasted vegetables, or toast, allow it to cool slightly.

CHAPTER 3
BREAKFASTS

Discover a world of Mediterranean-inspired breakfast recipes that are as beautiful as they are delicious. From savory to sweet, these dishes are sure to become your new morning favorites.

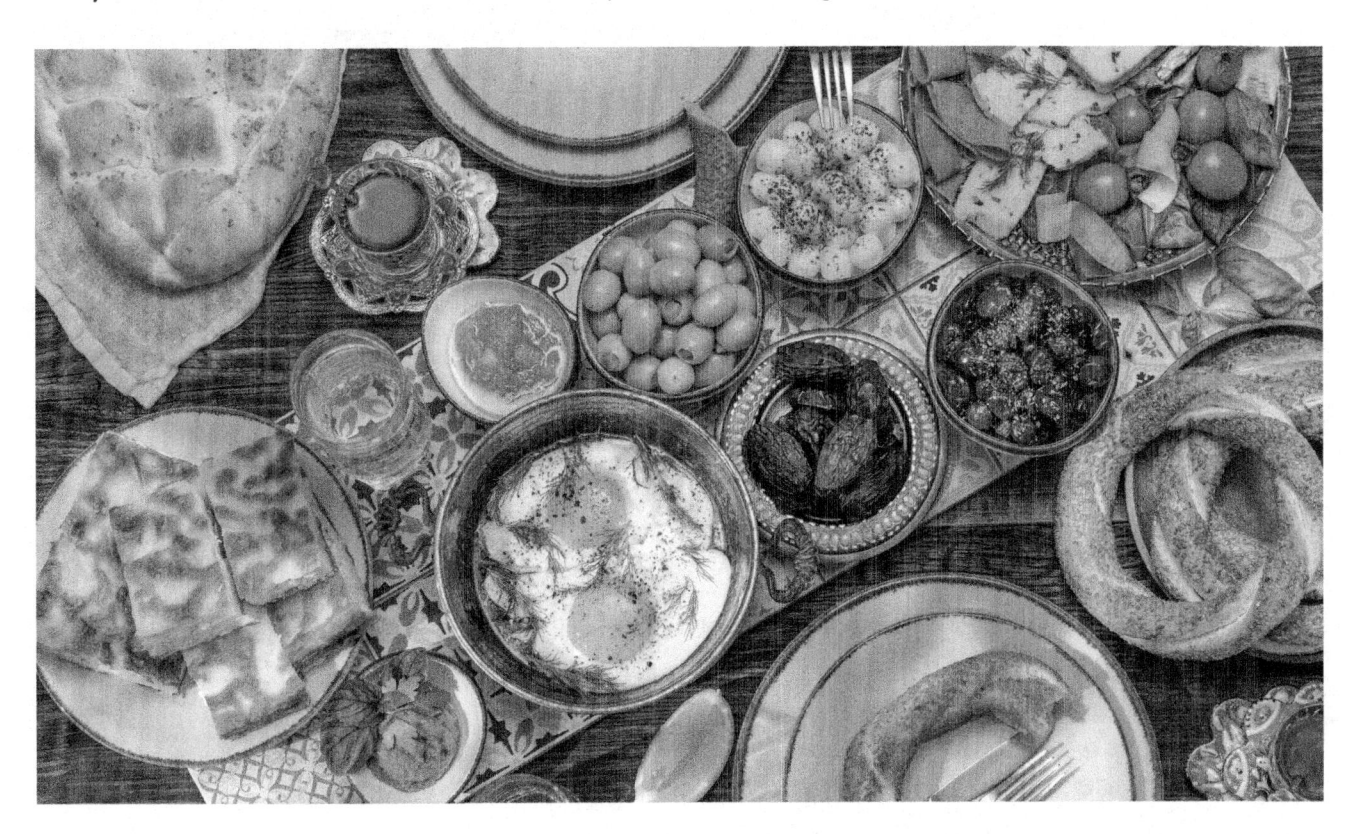

TIPS:

- Make your own yogurt, bread, or jams for a truly authentic Mediterranean breakfast experience.

- Enhance your breakfast experience with a cup of Greek coffee, Turkish tea, or a glass of freshly squeezed orange juice.

- Incorporate seasonal fruits and vegetables into your breakfast dishes for the freshest and most flavorful meals.

Savory Tomato-Basil Omelet

VEGETARIAN, GLUTEN FREE, DAIRY FREE
PREP TIME: 05 MIN **COOK TIME:** 05 MIN **SERVINGS:** 1
Calories: 200, Carbs: 3g, Fat: 15g, Protein: 12g, Fiber: 0g, Sodium: 160mg

- 2 large eggs
- 1 tbsp olive oil, divided
- 2 tbsp diced tomatoes
- 1 tbsp fresh basil, chopped
- 4 tsp finely minced shallots
- 1 pinch salt
- 1 pinch black pepper
- ¼ tsp dried oregano
- 1 pinch red chili flakes

1. Sauté shallots in ½ tbsp olive oil over low heat until softened. Add tomatoes, oregano, chili flakes, salt, and pepper; simmer until thickened.
2. Beat eggs with a pinch of salt and 1 tbsp water for a fluffier texture.
3. Heat the remaining olive oil in a skillet, pour in eggs, and cook until just set.
4. Spread the tomato mixture over one side, sprinkle with basil, and fold. Garnish with extra basil if desired.

Sweet Almond and Fig Barley with Vanilla and Coconut

VEGETARIAN, DAIRY FREE
PREP TIME: 05 MIN **COOK TIME:** 25 MIN **SERVINGS:** 2
Calories: 270, Carbs: 45g, Fat: 9g, Protein: 7g, Fiber: 5g, Sodium: 55mg

- ½ cup pearl barley
- 2 cups almond milk
- 3 dried figs, chopped
- 2 tbsp slivered almonds
- 1 tsp ground cinnamon
- ½ tsp vanilla extract
- 1 tbsp shredded coconut (unsweetened)
- 1 tsp maple syrup (optional for added sweetness)

1. Put almond milk and pearl barley in a saucepan.
2. Bring to a boil over medium heat, then lower the heat and simmer, stirring periodically, until the mixture is creamy and the barley is tender, 15 to 20 minutes.
3. Add dried figs, vanilla extract, and ground cinnamon.
4. Let the figs soften and incorporate into the porridge by continuing to simmer for a further two to three minutes.
5. Spoon the porridge into bowls, then sprinkle with shredded coconut and slivered almonds.
6. For a little sweetness, you can pour maple syrup on top if you'd like.
7. For a warm, cozy breakfast or snack, serve right away.

Greek Yogurt with Honey, Walnuts, and Spiced Raisin Syrup

VEGETARIAN, GLUTEN FREE
PREP TIME: 10 MIN **COOK TIME:** 05 MIN **SERVINGS:** 1
Calories: 195, Carbs: 19g, Fat: 9g, Protein: 9g, Fiber: 1g, Sodium: 30mg

- ½ cup plain Greek yogurt
- 1 tsp honey, plus ½ tsp for syrup
- 1 tbsp chopped walnuts
- 1 tbsp raisins
- 2 tbsp water
- 1 pinch ground cinnamon
- 1 pinch ground nutmeg

1. Put raisins, water, ½ tsp honey, and a pinch of ground cinnamon and nutmeg in a small pot.
2. Stirring occasionally, boil over low heat until the liquid reduces to a thick syrup and the raisins plump up, about 3 to 5 minutes.
3. Greek yogurt should be spooned into a serving bowl.
4. Evenly drizzle the yogurt with honey.
5. Over the yogurt, scatter chopped walnuts.
6. For extra taste, drizzle the warm spiced raisin syrup over the top.
7. Garnish with a last pinch of cinnamon and serve right away.

Mediterranean Scramble with Lemon Zest and Spinach

VEGETARIAN, GLUTEN FREE, DAIRY FREE
PREP TIME: 05 MIN **COOK TIME:** 10 MIN **SERVINGS:** 1
Calories: 175, Carbs: 2g, Fat: 14g, Protein: 10g, Fiber: 1g, Sodium: 120mg

- 2 large eggs
- 1 tbsp olive oil
- 2 tbsp diced bell peppers
- 2 tbsp chopped spinach
- ¼ tsp lemon zest
- 1 pinch dried oregano
- 1 tsp finely chopped sun-dried tomatoes (in olive oil)
- 1 pinch salt
- 1 pinch black pepper

1. Beat eggs with a pinch of salt until smooth.
2. Heat olive oil in a skillet over medium heat, sauté

bell peppers for 1 minute.
3. Add sun-dried tomatoes and spinach, cooking until softened, 1–2 minutes.
4. Stir in oregano, black pepper, and lemon zest, then pour in eggs.
5. Gently scramble eggs until just set.
6. Serve with a garnish of lemon zest or oregano

Lemon Herb Millet Porridge Garlic-Infused Oil

VEGETARIAN, GLUTEN FREE, DAIRY FREE
PREP TIME: 05 MIN **COOK TIME:** 15 MIN **SERVINGS:** 2
Calories: 190, Carbs: 34g, Fat: 5g, Protein: 5g, Fiber: 3g, Sodium: 10mg

- ½ cup millet
- 1½ cups water
- 1 tbsp olive oil, divided
- 1 tsp lemon zest
- 2 tsp chopped parsley
- ½ tsp minced garlic
- ½ tsp lemon juice

1. Rinse millet and cook in boiling water for 12–15 minutes until tender.
2. Sauté garlic in olive oil until fragrant.
3. Mix cooked millet with olive oil, lemon zest, juice, parsley, and garlic oil.
4. Season with salt and pepper, then serve..

Frittata

GLUTEN FREE
PREP TIME: 05 MIN **COOK TIME:** 10 MIN **SERVINGS:** 2
Calories: 150, Carbs: 3g, Fat: 11g, Protein: 10g, Fiber: 1g, Sodium: 120mg

- 4 large eggs
- ½ cup mixed vegetables (e.g., spinach, bell peppers, or zucchini), chopped
- 2 tbsp milk
- ¼ cup grated cheese (optional for a vegetarian version)
- 1 tbsp olive oil

1. In a bowl, whisk together the eggs, milk, and a pinch of salt and pepper until well combined.
2. Heat olive oil in a small non-stick skillet over medium heat. Add the chopped vegetables and sauté for 2–3 minutes until softened.
3. Pour the egg mixture over the vegetables and cook for 3–4 minutes until the edges begin to set.
4. If using cheese, sprinkle it on top. Transfer the skillet to the oven and broil for 2–3 minutes, or until the frittata is golden and cooked through.
5. Slice and serve immediately.

Orange and Pistachio Breakfast Bowl with Almond Flakes and Mint

VEGETARIAN, GLUTEN FREE, DAIRY FREE
PREP TIME: 05 MIN **COOK TIME:** 00 MIN **SERVINGS:** 2
Calories: 195, Carbs: 19g, Fat: 9g, Protein: 5g, Fiber: 3g, Sodium: 25mg

- 1 cup plain coconut yogurt
- 1 large orange, segmented
- 2 tbsp pistachios, chopped
- 1 tsp orange blossom water
- 1 tsp honey
- 1 tbsp slivered almonds (optional)
- 1 tsp fresh mint, finely chopped

1. Plain coconut yogurt should be split between two dishes.
2. Gently stir the yogurt after adding orange segmented.
3. Top with pistachios and honey.
4. Evenly distribute the orange segments on top of the yogurt.
5. For texture and freshness, sprinkle with fresh mint and slivered almonds.
6. Serve right away for a light and refreshing breakfast.

Spiced Sweet Potato & Date Delight

VEGETARIAN, GLUTEN FREE, DAIRY FREE
PREP TIME: 05 MIN **COOK TIME:** 00 MIN **SERVINGS:** 1
Calories: 240, Carbs: 36g, Fat: 9g, Protein: 4g, Fiber: 6g, Sodium: 20mg

- 1 small cooked sweet potato, mashed
- 2 dates, finely chopped
- 1 tsp maple syrup
- 1 pinch cinnamon
- 1 tbsp crushed walnuts
- 1 tsp almond butter

1. Combine the chopped dates and mashed sweet potato in a bowl.
2. Add cinnamon, maple syrup, and almond butter, and stir well to combine.
3. Serve warm, garnished with crumbled walnuts.

Homemade Labneh

VEGETARIAN, GLUTEN FREE
PREP TIME: 10 MIN **COOK TIME:** 20 MIN **SERVINGS:** 4
Calories: 110, Carbs: 4g, Fat: 8g, Protein: 6g, Fiber: 0g, Sodium: 150mg

- 2 cups plain Greek yogurt (full-fat works best)
- ½ tsp salt
- 1 tbsp olive oil
- ¼ tsp dried mint
- ¼ tsp sumac

1. In a mixing bowl, combine the Greek yogurt and salt. Stir well to ensure the salt is evenly distributed.
2. Line a fine mesh sieve with cheesecloth or a clean kitchen towel. Place the yogurt mixture into the cloth, then gather the edges and tie them securely.
3. Place the sieve over a bowl to catch the whey and refrigerate for 20 minutes to allow the yogurt to thicken into labneh.
4. After chilling, transfer the labneh to a serving plate. Drizzle olive oil on top and sprinkle with dried mint and sumac.
5. Serve immediately with bread, crackers, or vegetable sticks.

Simple Caprese Medley

VEGETARIAN, GLUTEN FREE
PREP TIME: 05 MIN **COOK TIME:** 00 MIN **SERVINGS:** 2
Calories: 220, Carbs: 8g, Fat: 19g, Protein: 9g, Fiber: 2g, Sodium: 180mg

- 2 medium heirloom tomatoes, sliced
- 4 slices fresh mozzarella
- 6 fresh basil leaves, torn
- 1 tbsp extra virgin olive oil
- 1 tsp lemon zest
- 1 tsp aged balsamic vinegar
- 1 tsp white truffle oil
- 1 tbsp pine nuts, toasted
- 1 pinch sea salt
- Freshly cracked black pepper, to taste

1. Arrange the heirloom tomatoes in a circle on a large serving platter after slicing them into thick, even slices.
2. Slices of tomato should be arranged alternately with thick rounds of fresh mozzarella.
3. Scatter the freshly torn basil leaves over the mozzarella and tomatoes.
4. To add a zesty, fresh touch to the dish, squeeze the lemon and sprinkle the zest on top.
5. Toast the pine nuts in a small pan over low heat for two to three minutes, stirring now and then, until aromatic and brown. Take off the heat and place aside.
6. Put balsamic vinegar and extra virgin olive oil in a small pot. To enhance the flavor and slightly decrease, simmer on low for two to three minutes.
7. Over the tomatoes and mozzarella, drizzle white truffle oil and the balsamic reduction.
8. To taste, add freshly cracked black pepper, toasted pine nuts, and a dash of salt.

Mediterranean Avocado and Nut Bowl with Lemon-Oregano Drizzle

VEGETARIAN, GLUTEN FREE, DAIRY FREE
PREP TIME: 05 MIN **COOK TIME:** 00 MIN **SERVINGS:** 1
Calories: 270, Carbs: 12g, Fat: 25g, Protein: 4g, Fiber: 7g, Sodium: 10mg

- ½ ripe avocado, diced
- ½ cup cherry tomatoes, halved
- 1 tbsp extra virgin olive oil
- 1 tbsp fresh lemon juice
- 1 tsp dried oregano
- 1 tbsp chopped almonds or walnuts (your choice)
- 1 tsp lemon zest
- Freshly cracked black pepper, to taste
- 1 tbsp pomegranate seeds (optional for extra flavor and color)

1. Cut the cherry tomatoes in half and dice the avocado. In a medium bowl, put them.
2. Chop the walnuts or almonds and reserve them for another time.
3. Sprinkle the lemon's zest over the avocado and tomatoes once it has been squeezed.
4. Stir slowly to blend the tastes after adding the lemon juice and extra virgin olive oil.
5. Top with freshly cracked black pepper and dried oregano.
6. For a delicious crunch, add chopped nuts and pomegranate seeds, if using.
7. Gently stir everything together and serve right away to bring out the flavors of the fresh Mediterranean.

Zaatar and Olive-Infused Gluten Free Pita

VEGETARIAN, GLUTEN FREE, DAIRY FREE
PREP TIME: 05 MIN **COOK TIME:** 05 MIN **SERVINGS:** 1
Calories: 220, Carbs: 24g, Fat: 12g, Protein: 3g, Fiber: 4g, Sodium: 180mg

- 1 gluten-free pita bread
- 1 tsp zaatar seasoning
- 1 tbsp extra virgin olive oil
- 2 tbsp Kalamata olives, chopped
- 1 tsp lemon zest
- 1 tbsp fresh parsley, finely chopped
- 1 pinch sea salt (optional, to taste)

1. The gluten-free pita should be heated in a dry skillet over medium heat for one to two minutes, turning once, until it is gently crisp on both sides.
2. While the pita is still warm, remove it from the skillet and drizzle it with extra virgin olive oil.
3. Evenly distribute the zaatar spices on the pita.
4. For a fragrant finish, sprinkle the pita with chopped Kalamata olives, lemon zest, and fresh parsley.
5. For more flavor depth, lightly season with sea salt (optional).
6. Cut into slices and serve right away.

Sunrise Quinoa Delight

VEGETARIAN, GLUTEN FREE
PREP TIME: 05 MIN **COOK TIME:** 15 MIN **SERVINGS:** 2
Calories: 270, Carbs: 41g, Fat: 10g, Protein: 6g, Fiber: 6g, Sodium: 15mg

- ½ cup cooked quinoa
- 2 tbsp raisins
- 2 tbsp chopped almonds
- 1 tsp ground cinnamon
- 1 tsp honey
- 1 tbsp chia seeds
- 1 tbsp shredded coconut
- 1 tsp orange zest

1. Put the cooked quinoa, ground cinnamon, sliced almonds, raisins, and coconut shreds in a bowl.
2. Pour the orange zest and honey over the mixture. Mix everything well.
3. Top with chia seeds for an extra omega-3 and fiber boost.
4. Savor it warm or at room temperature for a filling and stimulating breakfast with a Mediterranean flair.

Parsley Olive Tapenade on Rice Cakes

VEGETARIAN, GLUTEN FREE, DAIRY FREE
PREP TIME: 05 MIN **COOK TIME:** 00 MIN **SERVINGS:** 1
Calories: 180, Carbs: 20g, Fat: 9g, Protein: 3g, Fiber: 3g, Sodium: 220mg

- 2 gluten-free rice cakes
- 2 tbsp olive tapenade
- 1 tsp lemon zest
- ½ tsp dried thyme
- 1 pinch black pepper
- 1 tbsp chopped fresh parsley
- 1 tbsp chopped sun-dried tomatoes
- 1 tsp olive oil

1. Evenly cover the rice cakes with olive tapenade after placing them on a plate.
2. Over the tapenade, scatter chopped sun-dried tomatoes, dried thyme, lemon zest, and black pepper.
3. Garnish with fresh parsley and drizzle with olive oil.
4. Serve right away for a colorful, breakfast.

Cardamom-Spiced Barley and Caramelized Pear Medley

VEGETARIAN, DAIRY FREE
PREP TIME: 10 MIN **COOK TIME:** 20 MIN **SERVINGS:** 2
Calories: 280, Carbs: 42g, Fat: 4g, Protein: 6g, Fiber: 6g, Sodium: 20mg

- ½ cup pearl barley
- 1½ cups almond milk
- 1 ripe pear, diced
- 1 tsp vanilla extract
- 1 tsp ground cardamom
- Olive oil

1. In a saucepan, simmer almond milk and pearl barley over medium heat. Reduce heat and cook for 15-20 minutes until barley softens and absorbs the milk, creating a creamy texture.
2. In a skillet, sauté chopped pear with olive oil over medium heat for 5-7 minutes until golden and caramelized.
3. Stir vanilla extract and ground cardamom into the cooked barley, letting it infuse on low heat for 1-2 minutes.
4. Spoon the creamy barley into bowls, top with caramelized pears, and drizzle any pan syrup.
5. Garnish with honey or crushed pistachios before serving.

Mediterranean Stuffed Avocado Boats with Tomato, Olive & Herb Filling

VEGETARIAN, GLUTEN FREE, DAIRY FREE
PREP TIME: 05 MIN **COOK TIME:** 00 MIN **SERVINGS:** 1
Calories: 280, Carbs: 12g, Fat: 24g, Protein: 3g, Fiber: 8g, Sodium: 150mg

- 1 avocado, halved and pitted
- 2 tbsp diced cherry tomatoes
- 1 tbsp chopped kalamata olives
- 1 tsp lemon juice
- 1 pinch dried oregano
- 1 tsp extra virgin olive oil

1. Slice the avocado in half and remove the pit. Scoop out a small portion of the flesh to create space for the filling and set it aside for later use.
2. In a bowl, mix the chopped olives, cherry tomatoes, olive oil, oregano, and lemon juice until well combined.
3. Spoon the mixture into the hollowed-out avocado halves, filling them generously.
4. Garnish with a sprinkle of oregano or a drizzle of olive oil. Serve immediately.

Lemon Zucchini Quinoa Bowl with Herb-Infused Olive Oil

VEGETARIAN, GLUTEN FREE, DAIRY FREE
PREP TIME: 05 MIN
COOK TIME: 10 MIN (QUINOA PREPARED AHEAD)
SERVINGS: 2
Calories: 200, Carbs: 28g, Fat: 8g, Protein: 5g, Fiber: 4g, Sodium: 60mg

- 1 cup cooked quinoa
- ½ cup diced zucchini (raw or lightly sautéed for a softer texture)
- 1 tbsp fresh lemon juice
- 1 tbsp extra virgin olive oil (infused with fresh herbs)
- 1 tbsp chopped fresh mint or parsley

1. In a small bowl, combine olive oil with parsley or mint leaves. Let it infuse for a few minutes. Optionally, warm the oil gently for 1-2 minutes to enhance the herb aroma, then let it cool slightly.
2. In a medium bowl, mix diced zucchini with cooked quinoa. Keep the zucchini raw for a crisp texture or sauté it lightly with olive oil if you prefer it softer.
3. Drizzle the herb-infused olive oil and fresh lemon juice over the quinoa and zucchini. Stir well to ensure the flavors are evenly distributed.
4. Fold in freshly chopped parsley or mint, adding a vibrant and refreshing touch to the dish.
5. Serve immediately or refrigerate for a chilled, flavorful meal. Enjoy at room temperature or cold.

Garlic-Infused Tomato-Basil Crostini with Balsamic Glaze

VEGETARIAN, DAIRY FREE
PREP TIME: 05 MIN **COOK TIME:** 05 MIN **SERVINGS:** 2
Calories: 180, Carbs: 22g, Fat: 10g, Protein: 3g, Fiber: 3g, Sodium: 120mg

- 2 slices gluten-free bread, toasted
- 1 medium tomato, thinly sliced
- 1 tsp balsamic vinegar
- 2 tbsp extra virgin olive oil (infused with garlic)
- 4 fresh basil leaves, finely chopped
- 1 pinch sea salt

1. Heat the olive oil in a small pan over low heat. Be careful not to burn the garlic as you add one smashed clove and let it marinate for two to three minutes. Take off the heat and throw away the garlic. Put aside the olive oil that has been steeped.
2. Toast the gluten-free bread slices until they are as crispy as you like.
3. Evenly drizzle the toasted bread slices with the olive oil scented with garlic.
4. Spread the toast with the thinly sliced tomatoes. Add freshly chopped basil leaves and sea salt.
5. Drizzle the balsamic vinegar over the tomato and basil.
6. Savor it right away as savory breakfast.

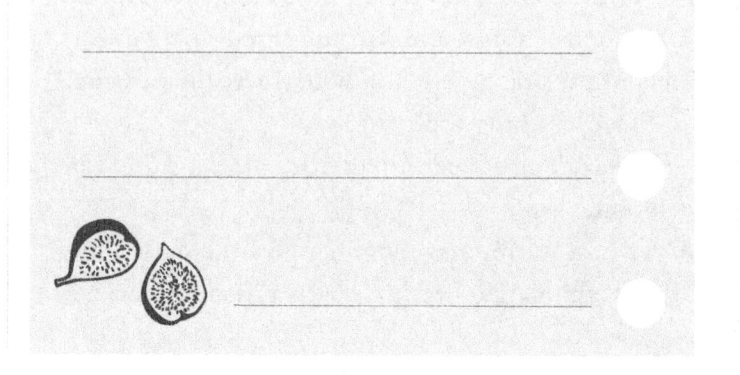

Mediterranean-Spiced Tofu Scramble with Bell Peppers and Tomato

VEGETARIAN, GLUTEN FREE, DAIRY FREE
PREP TIME: 05 MIN **COOK TIME:** 10 MIN **SERVINGS:** 2
Calories: 150, Carbs: 7g, Fat: 9g, Protein: 10g, Fiber: 2g, Sodium: 150mg

- 1 block (200g) firm tofu, crumbled
- ½ cup diced bell peppers
- ½ cup diced tomatoes
- 1 tbsp olive oil
- 1 tsp smoked paprika
- 1 tbsp chopped fresh parsley
- ½ tsp ground cumin
- 1 tbsp nutritional yeast (optional)

1. Heat the olive oil in a big skillet over medium heat. Cook bell peppers for two to three minutes, or until they are tender.
2. Cook for 5 minutes, or until the tofu starts to firm up a little, after adding the tomatoes and tofu.
3. Add ground cumin, smoked paprika, and nutritional yeast, if using, and stir. Allow the flavors to meld by cooking for a further three to four minutes.
4. Take off the heat, add some fresh parsley, and, if you want, tweak the seasoning with a touch of salt and pepper. Warm up and serve.

Bourekas

VEGETARIAN
PREP TIME: 10 MIN **COOK TIME:** 15 MIN **SERVINGS:** 4
Calories: 180, Carbs: 15g, Fat: 11g, Protein: 4g, Fiber: 1g, Sodium: 220mg

- 1 sheet puff pastry
- ½ cup feta cheese, crumbled
- ¼ cup spinach, chopped
- 1 egg, beaten
- ¼ tsp black sesame seeds

1. Preheat the oven to 375°F (190°C). Cut the puff pastry into 4 squares.
2. In a bowl, mix feta cheese and chopped spinach. Place a spoonful of the mixture in the center of each pastry square.
3. Fold each square into a triangle and seal the edges. Brush with beaten egg and sprinkle sesame seeds on top.
4. Bake for 15 minutes or until golden brown. Serve warm.

Pistachio Chia Banana Bowl

VEGETARIAN, GLUTEN FREE, DAIRY FREE
PREP TIME: 05 MIN **COOK TIME:** 00 MIN **SERVINGS:** 1
Calories: 230, Carbs: 35g, Fat: 12g, Protein: 5g, Fiber: 6g, Sodium: 5mg

- 1 ripe banana, sliced
- 1 tsp cinnamon
- 1 tsp honey (optional)
- 1 tbsp crushed pistachios
- 1 tbsp chia seeds
- 1 tbsp shredded coconut
- 1 tsp almond butter (optional)
- 1 pinch cinnamon (for garnish)

1. Arrange the banana slices in a serving bowl.
2. Drizzle with honey (if using) and almond butter (if using).
3. Sprinkle the ground cinnamon evenly over the banana slices.
4. Top with crushed pistachios, chia seeds, and shredded coconut.
5. Garnish with a final pinch of cinnamon before serving.

Cinnamon Figs & Seeds Porridge

VEGETARIAN, GLUTEN FREE, DAIRY FREE
PREP TIME: 05 MIN **COOK TIME:** 10 MIN **SERVINGS:** 2
Calories: 280, Carbs: 45g, Fat: 14g, Protein: 8g, Fiber: 10g, Sodium: 50mg

- 1 cup gluten-free rolled oats
- 2 cups almond milk
- 2 tbsp chopped dried figs
- 1 tsp honey
- 1 tsp ground cinnamon
- 1 tbsp chopped walnuts

1. In a small pot, combine almond milk and oats.
2. Cook over medium heat, stirring periodically for 5–7 minutes until the oats are tender.
3. Add cinnamon, honey, dried figs, walnuts, Stir well.
4. Continue cooking for an additional 2-3 minutes to ensure everything is heated through.
5. Serve warm, and garnish with extra walnuts or a drizzle of honey if desired.

Manakish with Feta and Ground Meat

PREP TIME: 15 MIN **COOK TIME:** 15 MIN **SERVINGS:** 4
Calories: 180, Carbs: 14g, Fat: 9g, Protein: 8g, Fiber: 1g, Sodium: 280mg

- 1 cup all-purpose flour
- ¼ cup water
- 2 tbsp olive oil
- 2 tbsp za'atar seasoning
- ¼ cup feta cheese, crumbled
- ¼ cup cooked ground meat (beef or lamb)
- ¼ tsp salt

1. In a mixing bowl, combine flour, water, olive oil, and salt. Knead until a soft dough forms.
2. Roll out the dough into a thin circle and place it on a greased baking sheet.
3. Evenly spread the za'atar seasoning over the dough. Sprinkle the crumbled feta cheese and cooked ground meat on top.
4. Bake at 400°F (200°C) for 12–15 minutes, or until the edges are golden brown and the toppings are slightly crisp.
5. Slice into portions and serve warm.

Pomegranate & Walnut Greek Yogurt Parfait

VEGETARIAN, GLUTEN FREE
PREP TIME: 05 MIN **COOK TIME:** 00 MIN **SERVINGS:** 1
Calories: 250, Carbs: 26g, Fat: 12g, Protein: 13g, Fiber: 6g, Sodium: 55mg

- ½ cup plain Greek yogurt
- 2 tbsp pomegranate seeds
- 1 tsp honey
- 1 tbsp chia seeds
- 2 tbsp diced fresh mango
- a pinch of ground cardamom

1. In a small bowl, spoon the Greek yogurt.
2. Layer with the diced mango, pomegranate seeds, and chia seed.
3. Drizzle honey over the top and sprinkle with sunflower seeds.
4. Garnish with a pinch of ground cardamom and serve.

Smoky Sweet Potato Breakfast Hash

VEGETARIAN, GLUTEN FREE, DAIRY FREE
PREP TIME: 10 MIN **COOK TIME:** 20 MIN **SERVINGS:** 2
Calories: 230, Carbs: 36g, Fat: 8g, Protein: 3g, Fiber: 7g, Sodium: 35mg

- 1 medium sweet potato, diced
- 1 tbsp olive oil
- 1 red bell pepper, diced
- 1 medium zucchini, diced
- 1 tbsp fresh cilantro, chopped
- 1 tsp smoked paprika

1. In a skillet, heat the olive oil over medium heat. Cook, stirring frequently, for 10 minutes after adding the cubed sweet potato.
2. Add the chopped zucchini and bell pepper, then the smoked paprika. Cook for a further five minutes or until everything is tender.
3. Before serving, garnish with chopped cilantro.

Sun-Kissed Chickpea and Avocado Breakfast Bowl

VEGETARIAN, GLUTEN FREE, DAIRY FREE
PREP TIME: 05 MIN **COOK TIME:** 00 MIN **SERVINGS:** 1
Calories: 250, Carbs: 30g, Fat: 12g, Protein: 7g, Fiber: 8g, Sodium: 150mg

- ½ cup canned chickpeas, rinsed and drained
- ¼ cup diced red bell pepper
- ¼ avocado, diced
- 1 tbsp parsley, finely chopped
- 1 tsp olive oil
- 1 tsp lemon juice
- 1 tbsp pomegranate seeds (optional)
- Smoked paprika for dashing

1. Add the diced avocado, parsley, red bell pepper, and chickpeas to a bowl.
2. Pour the lemon juice and olive oil over the mixture and gently toss to mix.
3. For more taste and color, sprinkle smoked paprika and pomegranate seeds on top.
4. Serve right away for a nutrient-dense, revitalizing breakfast.

Stuffed Sweet Potato with Avocado, Pomegranate & Toasted Seeds

VEGETARIAN, GLUTEN FREE, DAIRY FREE
PREP TIME: 05 MIN **COOK TIME:** 15 MIN **SERVINGS:** 1
Calories: 250, Carbs: 34g, Fat: 12g, Protein: 5g, Fiber: 8g, Sodium: 35mg

- 1 small sweet potato, baked
- ½ avocado, diced
- 2 tbsp pomegranate seeds
- 1 tsp olive oil
- 1 pinch cinnamon
- 1 tbsp toasted sunflower seeds (or pumpkin seeds)
- 1 tsp fresh lime juice

1. Slice the baked sweet potato in half and scoop out a small portion of the flesh, keeping the skin intact.
2. Mash the scooped sweet potato flesh with diced avocado until smooth.
3. Mix in lime juice, cinnamon, and olive oil for flavor.
4. Fill the sweet potato shells with the mashed mixture and top with pomegranate seeds and toasted sunflower seeds.
5. Serve immediately, optionally sprinkling with extra cinnamon.

Apple-Almond Delight Breakfast Bowl

VEGETARIAN, GLUTEN FREE, DAIRY FREE
PREP TIME: 05 MIN **COOK TIME:** 00 MIN **SERVINGS:** 1
Calories: 210, Carbs: 29g, Fat: 10g, Protein: 5g, Fiber: 5g, Sodium: 20mg

- 1 small apple, diced
- 2 tbsp almond butter
- 1 tsp ground cinnamon
- 1 tbsp chopped almonds
- 1 tbsp chia seeds
- 1 tbsp unsweetened shredded coconut

1. In a bowl, arrange the diced apple as the base.
2. Drizzle almond butter over the apples.
3. Sprinkle chopped almonds, ground cinnamon, chia seeds, and shredded coconut on top for added texture and flavor.
4. Stir gently to mix and enjoy!

Sun-Dried Tomato Chickpea Pancakes with Herbed Toppings

VEGETARIAN, GLUTEN FREE, DAIRY FREE
PREP TIME: 05 MIN **COOK TIME:** 10 MIN **SERVINGS:** 2
Calories: 230, Carbs: 30g, Fat: 9g, Protein: 9g, Fiber: 6g, Sodium: 180mg

- 1 cup chickpea flour
- ¾ cup water
- 1 tbsp olive oil
- 1 tsp dried oregano
- 1 pinch sea salt
- 1 tsp garlic powder
- 1 tbsp fresh parsley, chopped
- 1 tbsp sun-dried tomatoes, finely chopped
- 1 tbsp tahini (for drizzling)

1. Chickpea flour, water, olive oil, sea salt, oregano, garlic powder, parsley, and sun-dried tomatoes should all be combined in a bowl. The batter is formed by whisking until smooth.
2. Add a little olive oil to a nonstick skillet and heat it over medium heat. To make little pancakes, pour batter into the pan.
3. Cook each pancake until golden and crispy, 2 to 3 minutes per side.
4. If desired, top the warm pancakes with additional chopped parsley and tahini.

Tropical Avocado Mango Bowl

VEGETARIAN, GLUTEN FREE, DAIRY FREE
PREP TIME: 05 MIN **COOK TIME:** 00 MIN **SERVINGS:** 1
Calories: 210, Carbs: 22g, Fat: 15g, Protein: 5g, Fiber: 8g, Sodium: 10mg

- ½ avocado, diced
- ½ cup mango chunks
- 1 tbsp lime juice
- 1 tbsp chopped cilantro
- 1 pinch chili flakes (optional)
- 1 tbsp sunflower seeds
- 1 tbsp shredded coconut
- 1 tbsp hemp seeds

1. Put the diced mango and avocado in a bowl.
2. Sprinkle with chopped cilantro and drizzle with lime juice.
3. If desired, add chili flakes for a touch of spiciness.
4. Top with sunflower seeds, shredded coconut, and hemp seeds for added texture and nutrition.

CHAPTER 4

APPETIZERS, MEZE, TAPAS, SMALL PLATES

Embark on a culinary journey through the Mediterranean, where small plates reign supreme. From the bustling tapas bars of Spain to the vibrant mezze platters of the Middle East, these bite-sized delights are designed to tantalize your taste buds and ignite your appetite.

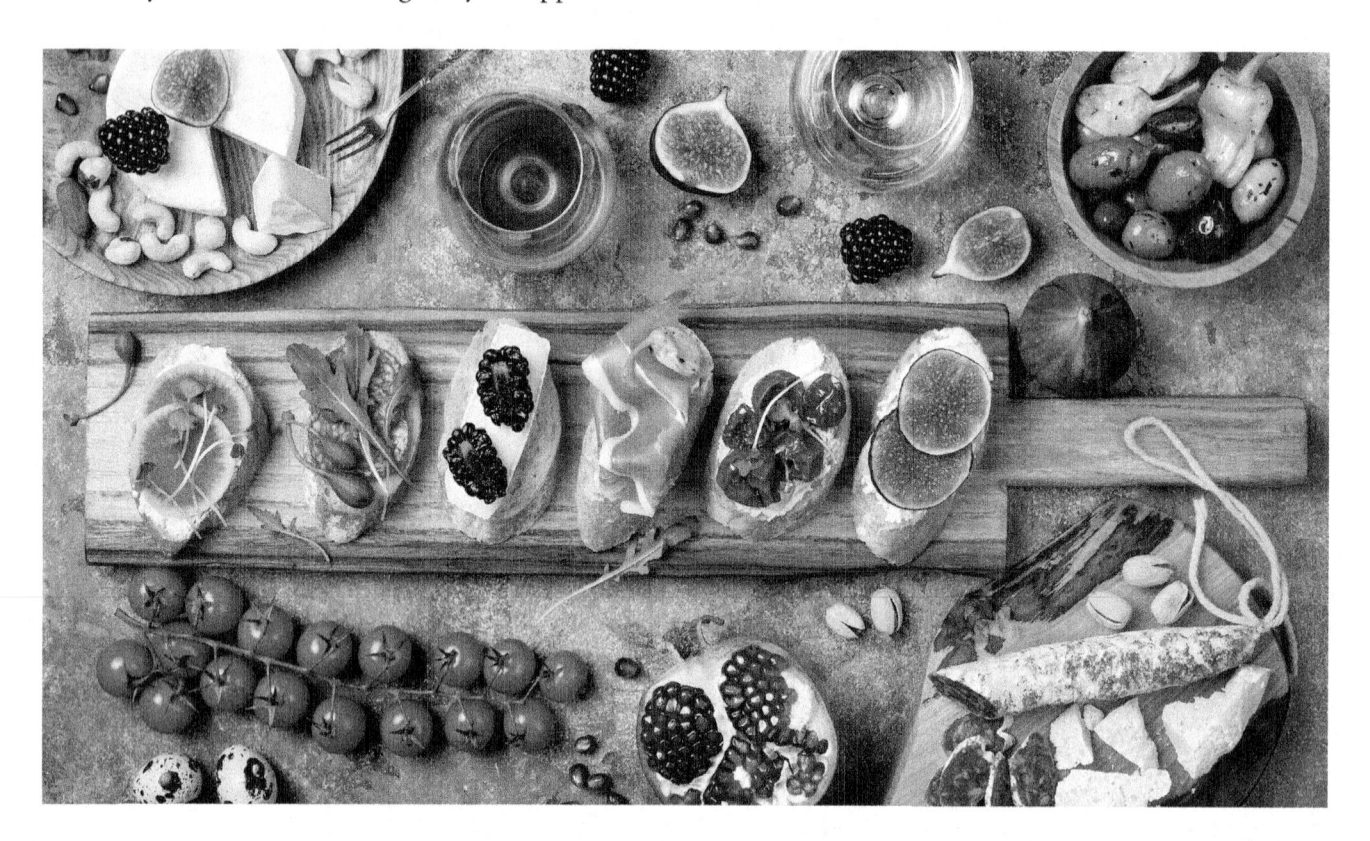

TIPS:

- A well-curated platter should offer a harmonious blend of flavors. Consider pairing sweet with savory, crunchy with creamy, and spicy with mild.

- Consider pairing your appetizers with complementary beverages, such as wine, beer, or cocktails.

- Engage your guests by incorporating interactive elements, such as DIY stations for tacos, bruschetta, or sushi.

Spiced Mini Peppers with Hummus and Herbs

VEGETARIAN, GLUTEN FREE
PREP TIME: 10 MIN **COOK TIME:** 05 MIN **SERVINGS:** 4
Calories: 110, Carbs: 8g, Fat: 6g, Protein: 3g, Fiber: 3g, Sodium: 150mg

- **12 mini sweet peppers, halved and deseeded**
- **½ cup hummus**
- **1 tbsp fresh dill, chopped**
- **1 tbsp fresh parsley, chopped**
- **1 tsp olive oil**
- **1 tsp lemon zest**
- **1 tbsp toasted sesame seeds**

1. Using a spoon or tiny knife, smooth the top of the hummus before spooning it into each mini pepper half.
2. For a zesty, fresh touch, sprinkle the stuffed peppers with chopped parsley, dill, and lemon zest.
3. Heat the olive oil in a small skillet over medium heat. For a deeper taste, drizzle the filled peppers with the heated oil.
4. For a nutty crunch, add roasted sesame seeds as a garnish. Serve right away.

Crispy Za'atar Chickpeas with Garlic

VEGETARIAN, GLUTEN FREE, DAIRY FREE
PREP TIME: 05 MIN **COOK TIME:** 10 MIN **SERVINGS:** 4
Calories: 120, Carbs: 18g, Fat: 4g, Protein: 5g, Fiber: 4g, Sodium: 160mg

- **1 can (15 oz) chickpeas, drained and rinsed**
- **1 tbsp olive oil**
- **1 tsp za'atar seasoning**
- **½ tsp garlic powder**
- **¼ tsp sea salt**
- **½ tsp smoked paprika**
- **1 tbsp fresh parsley, chopped**

1. Place a skillet on a medium heat source.
2. Combine the drained chickpeas, sea salt, smoked paprika (if using), garlic powder, olive oil, and za'atar in a bowl and toss until well coated.
3. Stirring often, add the seasoned chickpeas to the skillet and cook until golden and crispy, about 10 minutes.
4. Take off the heat and add some freshly cut parsley as a garnish. Serve right away for a crispy, toasty snack.

Basil-Infused Tomato Crostini

VEGETARIAN, DAIRY FREE
PREP TIME: 10 MIN **COOK TIME:** 05 MIN **SERVINGS:** 6
Calories: 100, Carbs: 14g, Fat: 4g, Protein: 2g, Fiber: 1g, Sodium: 130mg

- **1 baguette, sliced into 12 pieces**
- **2 tbsp olive oil**
- **1 cup cherry tomatoes, finely diced**
- **¼ cup Kalamata olives, chopped**
- **1 tbsp balsamic vinegar**
- **1 tbsp fresh basil, chopped (for garnish)**
- **1 tsp garlic powder (optional)**

1. Set the oven's temperature to 375°F. Place the baguette slices on a baking pan after brushing them with olive oil. Toast in the oven until golden and crispy, about 5 minutes.
2. Combine the chopped Kalamata olives, balsamic vinegar, chopped cherry tomatoes, and optional garlic powder in a bowl. Mix thoroughly to incorporate.
3. Spoon the tomato-olive mixture onto each slice of baguette after it has toasted. If desired, garnish with fresh basil. Serve right away.

Zesty Cucumber Feta Bites

VEGETARIAN, GLUTEN FREE
PREP TIME: 10 MIN **COOK TIME:** 00 MIN **SERVINGS:** 4
Calories: 90, Carbs: 3g, Fat: 6g, Protein: 3g, Fiber: 0g, Sodium: 120mg

- **1 cucumber, sliced into 12 rounds**
- **½ cup crumbled feta cheese**
- **1 tbsp plain Greek yogurt**
- **1 tsp lemon juice**
- **1 tsp fresh dill, chopped**
- **1 tbsp chopped mint**
- **1 tsp olive oil (optional for drizzling)**

1. In a small bowl, combine feta cheese, Greek yogurt, lemon juice, chopped dill, and chopped mint. Stir until smooth and well combined.
2. Spoon a generous dollop of the feta mixture onto each cucumber slice.
3. Garnish with extra dill and mint, and drizzle with olive oil if desired.
4. Serve immediately for a refreshing and creamy bite.

Spinach & Pine Nut Puff Rolls

VEGETARIAN, DAIRY FREE
PREP TIME: 10 MIN **COOK TIME:** 05 MIN **SERVINGS:** 6
Calories: 160, Carbs: 12g, Fat: 9g, Protein: 2g, Fiber: 1g, Sodium: 110mg

- 1 sheet of puff pastry, thawed
- 1 cup fresh spinach, chopped
- 2 tbsp pine nuts, toasted
- 1 tbsp olive oil
- 1 tsp ground nutmeg
- ¼ cup grated Parmesan cheese (optional)

1. Preheat the oven to 400°F (200°C).
2. Heat the olive oil in a pan over medium heat. Add the chopped spinach and ground nutmeg, and sauté until the spinach wilts. Let it cool slightly.
3. Unroll the puff pastry sheet, spread the spinach mixture evenly on top, and sprinkle toasted pine nuts and grated Parmesan cheese (optional) over it.
4. Carefully roll the puff pastry into a log and slice it into 1-inch rounds.
5. Arrange the slices on a baking sheet and bake for 10 to 12 minutes or until golden and puffed.
6. Serve warm and enjoy!

Balsamic Marinated Mushrooms with Fresh Herbs

VEGETARIAN, GLUTEN FREE, DAIRY FREE
PREP TIME: 10 MIN **COOK TIME:** 05 MIN **SERVINGS:** 4
Calories: 60, Carbs: 5g, Fat: 4g, Protein: 2g, Fiber: 1g, Sodium: 20mg

- 2 cups button mushrooms, cleaned
- 2 tbsp balsamic vinegar
- 1 tbsp olive oil
- 1 clove garlic, minced
- 1 tsp dried oregano
- 1 tbsp fresh parsley, chopped
- 1 tsp lemon zest

1. Heat the olive oil in a skillet over medium heat and cook the mushrooms for 3 minutes.
2. Add the oregano, garlic, balsamic vinegar, and lemon zest. Cook for an additional 2 minutes, or until the mushrooms are soft and tender.
3. Stir in fresh parsley and cook for another minute.
4. Serve warm or at room temperature.

Herbed Labneh Balls with Lemon & Pistachios

VEGETARIAN, GLUTEN FREE
PREP TIME: 10 MIN (PLUS 8 HOURS FOR STRAINING YOGURT) **COOK TIME:** 00 MIN **SERVINGS:** 6
Calories: 90, Carbs: 3g, Fat: 4g, Protein: 6g, Fiber: 0g, Sodium: 140mg

- 2 cups plain Greek yogurt
- 1 tsp sea salt
- 1 tbsp olive oil
- 1 tbsp lemon zest
- 2 tbsp chopped pistachios
- 1 tbsp honey
- 1 tsp lemon juice

1. Over a bowl, strain yogurt in a sieve lined with cheesecloth and refrigerate for 8 hours.
2. Once strained, add the salt, lemon zest, honey, and lemon juice to the yogurt and mix well.
3. Form the yogurt mixture into small balls and roll them in chopped pistachios for added crunch.
4. Drizzle with olive oil and serve with fresh vegetables or gluten-free crackers.

Stuffed Grape Leaves with Quinoa & Veggies

VEGETARIAN, GLUTEN FREE, DAIRY FREE
PREP TIME: 10 MIN **COOK TIME:** 10 MIN **SERVINGS:** 4
Calories: 100, Carbs: 12g, Fat: 2g, Protein: 3g, Fiber: 2g, Sodium: 180mg

- 12 grape leaves, jarred or fresh
- 1 cup cooked quinoa
- ½ cup shredded carrot
- ½ cup cucumber, finely diced
- 2 tbsp lemon juice
- 1 clove garlic, minced

1. Add the cooked quinoa, chopped cucumber, minced garlic, lemon juice, and shredded carrot to a bowl. Stir thoroughly.
2. Flatten the grape leaves, clean them (or blanch them if they are new), and then pat dry.
3. Roll firmly after placing 1 tablespoon of the quinoa mixture on each leaf and folding in the sides.
4. Put the rolls in a steamer basket, fill it with water, and steam them for five minutes to make them soft.
5. Before serving, remove and allow to cool somewhat. Warm or room temperature, enjoy.

Paprika Deviled Egg

VEGETARIAN, GLUTEN FREE
PREP TIME: 10 MIN **COOK TIME:** 10 MIN **SERVINGS:** 4
Calories: 100, Carbs: 2g, Fat: 6g, Protein: 7g, Fiber: 0g, Sodium: 120mg

- 6 large eggs
- 3 tbsp plain Greek yogurt
- 1 tbsp Kalamata olives, finely chopped
- 1 tsp olive oil
- ½ tsp paprika
- 1 tbsp capers, finely chopped
- 1 tsp fresh lemon juice

1. Boil eggs for 10 minutes, cool under cold water, and peel.
2. Remove yolks, mash with a fork, and mix with yogurt, olives, olive oil, capers, and lemon juice.
3. Fill egg whites with the mixture.
4. Garnish with paprika, capers, or olives.
5. Serve immediately or chill for 30 minutes.

Warm Feta with Honey and Thyme

VEGETARIAN, GLUTEN FREE
PREP TIME: 05 MIN **COOK TIME:** 05 MIN **SERVINGS:** 4
Calories: 150, Carbs: 3g, Fat: 9g, Protein: 5g, Fiber: 0g, Sodium: 310mg

- 200g (7 oz) block of feta cheese
- 1 tbsp honey
- 1 tsp fresh thyme leaves
- 1 tsp olive oil
- Pinch of black pepper
- 2 tbsp chopped walnuts
- 1 tbsp pomegranate seeds
- 1 tbsp balsamic vinegar

1. In a skillet, heat the olive oil over medium heat.
2. The feta block should be warm and starting to become golden after 2 to 3 minutes on each side of the skillet.
3. Drizzle with honey and garnish with fresh thyme leaves and a pinch of black pepper.
4. Drizzle the warm feta with balsamic vinegar for a tart finish, and add chopped walnuts and pomegranate seeds.
5. Serve right away with gluten-free crackers or slices of cucumber for crispness.

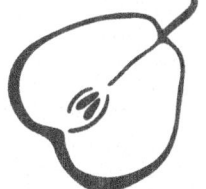

Grilled Eggplant with Pine Nuts

VEGETARIAN, GLUTEN FREE, DAIRY FREE
PREP TIME: 10 MIN **COOK TIME:** 10 MIN **SERVINGS:** 4
Calories: 80, Carbs: 6g, Fat: 5g, Protein: 1g, Fiber: 3g, Sodium: 5mg

- 2 medium eggplants, sliced lengthwise
- 2 tbsp olive oil
- 1 clove garlic, minced
- 1 tbsp lemon juice
- 1 tsp fresh parsley, chopped
- 1 tbsp tahini
- 1 tbsp pine nuts, toasted

1. Preheat the grill or grill pan to medium-high. Slice the eggplants lengthwise into ½ inch thick pieces, season with salt, and drizzle with olive oil. Grill for 3–4 minutes on each side until tender and marked.
2. In a small bowl, mix lemon juice and minced garlic. Let sit to blend flavors.
3. Once grilled, place the eggplants on a serving plate and drizzle with the garlic-lemon mixture.
4. Toast pine nuts in a small pan over medium heat for 1–2 minutes until aromatic and browned.
5. Top the eggplants with toasted pine nuts, drizzle with tahini, and garnish with chopped parsley.

Spinach and Feta Phyllo Triangles

VEGETARIAN
PREP TIME: 15 MIN **COOK TIME:** 10 MIN **SERVINGS:** 6
Calories: 150, Carbs: 10g, Fat: 9g, Protein: 5g, Fiber: 1g, Sodium: 160mg

- 1 cup fresh spinach, chopped
- ½ cup crumbled feta cheese
- 1 tbsp olive oil
- 6 sheets phyllo dough
- 1 tbsp melted butter
- ¼ cup ricotta cheese

1. Heat olive oil in a skillet, cook spinach for 2-3 minutes until wilted, then cool.
2. Mix crumbled feta, ricotta, and spinach in a bowl.
3. Brush phyllo dough with melted butter, layering sheets.
4. Slice dough into 3 strips, add filling, and fold into triangles.
5. Place triangles on a baking sheet, brush with butter, and bake at 375°F (190°C) for 10 minutes until golden.
6. Cool for a few minutes before serving.

Cucumber and Mint Gazpacho Shots

VEGETARIAN, GLUTEN FREE, DAIRY FREE
PREP TIME: 10 MIN **COOK TIME:** 10 MIN **SERVINGS:** 4
Calories: 80, Carbs: 5g, Fat: 3g, Protein: 1g, Fiber: 1g, Sodium: 50mg

- 2 large cucumbers, peeled and chopped
- 1 cup plain almond milk
- 1 clove garlic
- 1 tbsp olive oil
- 2 tbsp fresh mint leaves
- ½ cup avocado, peeled and chopped
- 1 tbsp lemon juice

1. Add the avocado, olive oil, garlic, diced cucumbers, and almond milk to a blender. Blend until it's smooth.
2. To ensure even mixing, add the lemon juice and blend for ten more seconds.
3. Before serving, place the gazpacho in the fridge to chill for at least half an hour.
4. Transfer the cooled soup into bowls or little glasses. For a refreshing touch, sprinkle some fresh mint leaves on top. Enjoy right away after serving.

Sun-Dried Tomato and Olive Tapenade

VEGETARIAN, GLUTEN FREE, DAIRY FREE
PREP TIME: 05 MIN **COOK TIME:** 00 MIN **SERVINGS:** 4
Calories: 80, Carbs: 3g, Fat: 7g, Protein: 1g, Fiber: 1g, Sodium: 200mg

- ½ cup sun-dried tomatoes in oil, drained
- ¼ cup Kalamata olives, pitted
- 1 clove garlic
- 2 tbsp olive oil
- 1 tsp capers
- ¼ cup roasted red peppers

1. In a food processor, combine the sun-dried tomatoes, Kalamata olives, minced garlic, capers, roasted red peppers. Pulse a few times until the mixture is well combined but still slightly chunky.
2. Slowly drizzle in the olive oil while continuing to pulse until the tapenade reaches a thick, spreadable consistency.
3. Add the lemon juice and pulse again to incorporate.
4. Transfer the tapenade to a serving dish, drizzle with a bit more olive oil if desired.
5. Serve with fresh vegetable sticks, gluten-free crackers,

Marinated Artichokes and Olives Medley

VEGETARIAN, GLUTEN FREE, DAIRY FREE
PREP TIME: 05 MIN **COOK TIME:** 00 MIN **SERVINGS:** 4
Calories: 110, Carbs: 3g, Fat: 7g, Protein: 1g, Fiber: 2g, Sodium: 240mg

- 1 cup artichoke hearts, drained
- ½ cup Kalamata olives, pitted
- 2 tbsp olive oil
- 1 tbsp lemon juice
- 1 tsp dried oregano
- 1 tbsp capers, drained
- ½ cup roasted red peppers, sliced
- ¼ cup diced red onion

1. In a medium-sized mixing bowl, start by draining the Kalamata olives and artichoke hearts.
2. To the bowl, add the diced red onion, capers, and roasted red peppers.
3. To make the dressing, combine the olive oil, lemon juice, and dried oregano in a different small bowl.
4. Drizzle the olive and artichoke combination with the dressing. Make sure all the ingredients are evenly covered by gently tossing to incorporate.
5. To give the flavors time to marinade and combine, cover the bowl with plastic wrap and place it in the refrigerator for at least ten minutes.
6. To serve as an appetizer, atop a salad, or as a garnish for gluten-free crackers, gently toss the marinated mixture one last time.

Spinach & Chickpea Bruschetta

VEGETARIAN, DAIRY FREE
PREP TIME: 10 MIN **COOK TIME:** 05 MIN **SERVINGS:** 6
Calories: 110, Carbs: 14g, Fat: 4g, Protein: 3g, Fiber: 2g, Sodium: 120mg

- 1 cup canned chickpeas, drained and rinsed
- 1 cup fresh spinach, chopped
- 1 clove garlic, minced
- 2 tbsp olive oil
- 6 slices of crusty bread or gluten-free bread
- 1 tbsp tahini
- ½ lemon, juiced

1. In a large skillet, heat the olive oil over medium heat to start. Add the minced garlic and cook until fragrant, about 1 minute.
2. Stir occasionally after adding the chopped spinach

to the pan. Cook until the spinach is wilted, 2 to 3 minutes.

3. After draining, add the chickpeas to the skillet and cook for a further two minutes, or until they are thoroughly heated and have a small crispy edge.
4. To uniformly coat the chickpeas and spinach, stir in the tahini and lemon juice. Give the mixture a minute to cool.
5. Toast the bread pieces in the meantime until they are crisp and brown.
6. Spoon the chickpea-spinach mixture onto each slice of bread as soon as it's ready.
7. Serve right away, with a bit more lemon juice or a drizzle of olive oil if desired

Roasted Cauliflower and Chickpea Bowl

VEGETARIAN, GLUTEN FREE, DAIRY FREE
PREP TIME: 10 MIN **COOK TIME:** 25 MIN **SERVINGS:** 4
Calories: 180, Carbs: 25g, Fat: 4g, Protein: 6g, Fiber: 7g, Sodium: 240mg

- 1 medium cauliflower, cut into florets
- 1 cup canned chickpeas, drained and rinsed
- 1 tbsp olive oil
- 1 tbsp lemon juice
- 1 tsp cumin
- 1 tsp paprika
- ½ cup cherry tomatoes, halved
- 2 tbsp fresh parsley, chopped

1. Set the oven's temperature to 400°F, or 200°C.
2. Add a touch of salt and pepper, cumin, paprika, and olive oil to the chickpeas and cauliflower florets. Evenly distribute them on a baking pan.
3. Roast for 20 to 25 minutes, stirring halfway through, until the chickpeas are crispy and the cauliflower is golden.
4. Take it out of the oven and let it to cool a little.
5. Add the roasted cauliflower and chickpeas, lemon juice, chopped parsley, and halved cherry tomatoes to a large bowl.
6. Serve warm or room temperature after gently tossing to blend.

Lentil and Veggie Lettuce Wraps

VEGETARIAN, GLUTEN FREE, DAIRY FREE
PREP TIME: 10 MIN **COOK TIME:** 00 MIN **SERVINGS:** 4
Calories: 100, Carbs: 12g, Fat: 3g, Protein: 5g, Fiber: 4g, Sodium: 10mg

- 1 cup cooked green lentils
- 1 cup mixed fresh herbs (parsley, mint, cilantro), chopped
- 1 tbsp lemon juice
- 1 tbsp olive oil
- 1 small cucumber, diced
- ½ cup cherry tomatoes, diced
- 1 small red onion, finely chopped
- Lettuce leaves for wrapping

1. Put the cooked lentils, lemon juice, olive oil, and chopped herbs in a big bowl.
2. Stir the mixture thoroughly after adding the red onion, cherry tomatoes, and chopped cucumber.
3. Form little cups by scooping the mixture onto each lettuce leaf.
4. Serve right away or store in the refrigerator for later.

Fresh Cucumber & Tomato Avocado Toast

VEGETARIAN, DAIRY FREE
PREP TIME: 10 MIN **COOK TIME:** 00 MIN **SERVINGS:** 6
Calories: 120, Carbs: 14g, Fat: 7g, Protein: 2g, Fiber: 1g, Sodium: 150mg

- 1 cup diced cherry tomatoes
- ½ cup diced cucumber
- 1 ripe avocado, diced
- 2 tbsp olive oil
- 1 tbsp balsamic vinegar
- 6 slices crusty bread or gluten-free bread

1. Toast the bread slices until they are crispy and golden brown. Let it cool a little.
2. Add the diced avocado, cucumber, and tomatoes to a medium bowl.
3. Toss gently until all ingredients are fully combined after adding the balsamic vinegar and olive oil to the bowl.
4. For optimal flavor and texture, spoon the mixture onto each slice of toasted bread and serve right away.

Cucumber and Feta Rolls with Lemon Zest

VEGETARIAN, GLUTEN FREE
PREP TIME: 10 MIN **COOK TIME:** 10 MIN **SERVINGS:** 4
Calories: 70, Carbs: 3g, Fat: 5g, Protein: 3g, Fiber: 0g, Sodium: 100mg

- **1 large cucumber**
- **½ cup crumbled feta cheese**
- **1 tbsp fresh dill, chopped**
- **1 tbsp olive oil**
- **1 tsp lemon zest**
- **¼ cup roasted red pepper, finely chopped**
- **2 tbsp pine nuts, toasted**
- **1 tbsp honey**

1. Cut the cucumber into thin, even strips lengthwise using a mandoline. To get rid of extra moisture, place the slices on a paper towel.
2. Combine the feta crumbles, lemon zest, olive oil, dill, and roasted red pepper in a bowl and stir until thoroughly blended.
3. Add a little honey for sweetness and gently mix in the toasted pine nuts.
4. Put a tiny dollop of the feta mixture on one end of each slice of cucumber. Using a toothpick if needed, firmly roll the cucumber slices around the filling.
5. For optimal texture, arrange the rolls on a dish and serve cold or room temperature.

Stuffed Mushrooms with Sun-Dried Tomato and Feta

VEGETARIAN, GLUTEN FREE
PREP TIME: 10 MIN **COOK TIME:** 10 MIN **SERVINGS:** 6
Calories: 60, Carbs: 2g, Fat: 4g, Protein: 3g, Fiber: 1g, Sodium: 110mg

- **12 large button mushrooms, stems removed**
- **½ cup crumbled feta cheese**
- **¼ cup sun-dried tomatoes, chopped**
- **1 tbsp olive oil**
- **1 tsp dried oregano**
- **2 tbsp Kalamata olives, chopped**
- **2 tbsp roasted red pepper, chopped**

1. Turn the oven on to 375°F, or 190°C. Put parchment paper on a baking pan.
2. Crumbled feta, chopped sun-dried tomatoes, olive oil, oregano, Kalamata olives, and roasted red pepper should all be combined in a mixing dish. Mix the ingredients until they are fully blended.
3. To make sure the mixture is packed firmly, carefully spoon it into the hollowed-out mushroom caps while applying a little pressure.
4. Make sure the stuffed mushrooms are not touching one another when you arrange them on the baking sheet that has been prepared.
5. The stuffed mushrooms should be browned and the filling should be just melted after 10 minutes of baking in a preheated oven.
6. Before serving warm, take it out of the oven and allow it to cool for a minute.

Crispy Sweet Potato and Chickpea Patties

VEGETARIAN, GLUTEN FREE
PREP TIME: 10 MIN **COOK TIME:** 10 MIN **SERVINGS:** 4
Calories: 130, Carbs: 10g, Fat: 8g, Protein: 6g, Fiber: 2g, Sodium: 180mg

- **2 medium sweet potatoes, grated and excess moisture squeezed out**
- **½ cup cooked chickpeas, mashed**
- **¼ cup gluten-free breadcrumbs**
- **1 egg**
- **2 tbsp chopped fresh cilantro and parsley**
- **1 tbsp olive oil**
- **1 tbsp lemon zest**
- **½ tsp ground cumin**
- **Salt and black pepper to taste**

1. Mix grated sweet potatoes, mashed chickpeas, egg, breadcrumbs, herbs, lemon zest, cumin, salt, and pepper.
2. Heat olive oil in a skillet over medium heat.
3. Form the mixture into small patties and cook for 3-4 minutes on each side until golden and crispy.
4. Drain excess oil on paper towels and serve warm with extra herbs or lemon juice.

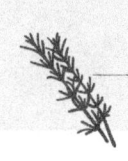

CHAPTER 5
SOUPS

Warm up your senses and nourish your soul with a comforting bowl of soup. From hearty stews to light broths, this chapter explores a diverse range of soups inspired by the rich culinary traditions of the Mediterranean.

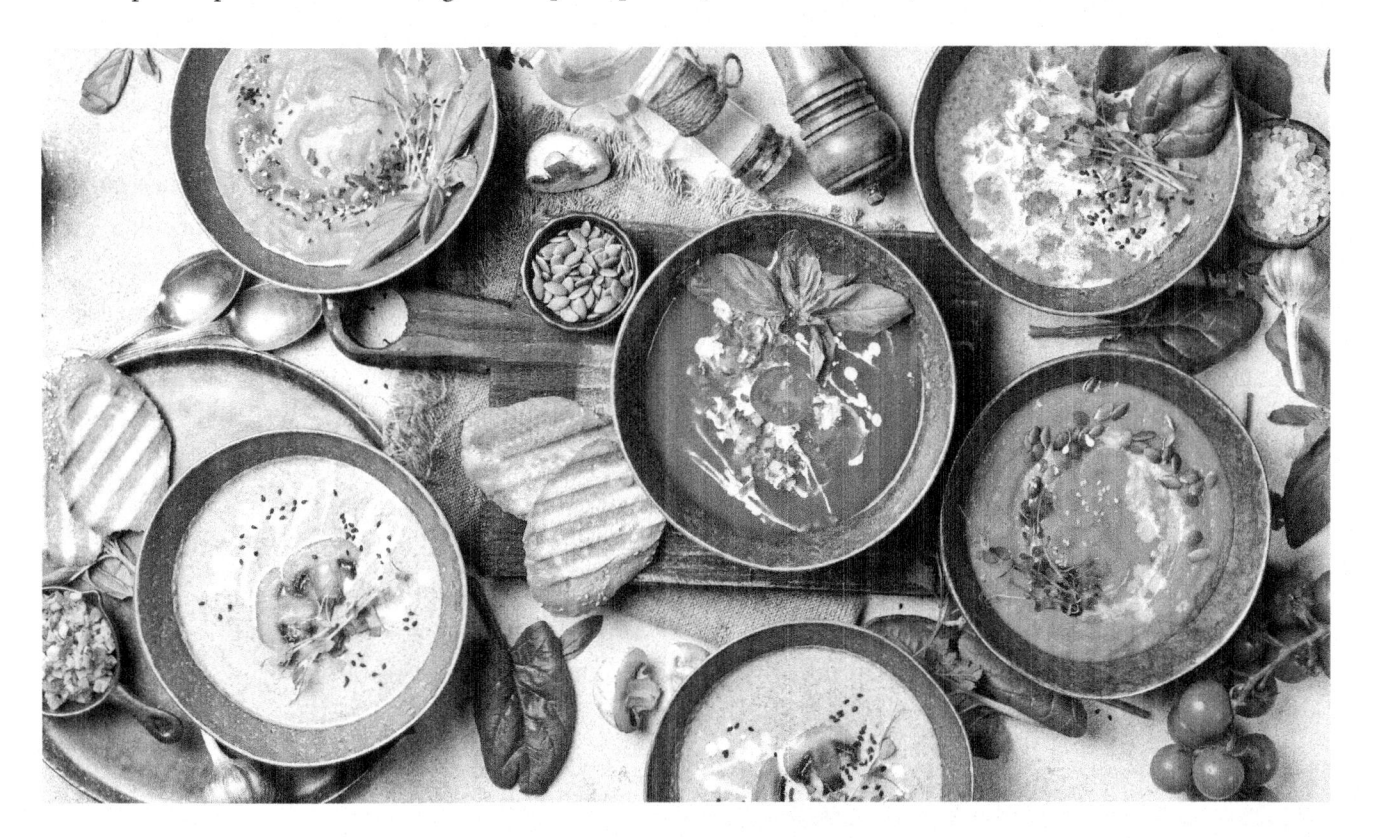

> **TIPS:**
>
> - Let your broth simmer for longer to develop a richer flavor.
>
> - A simple garnish can elevate a bowl of soup. Consider adding fresh herbs, grated cheese, croutons, or a drizzle of olive oil.
>
> - Serve your soup with a crusty loaf of bread, grilled cheese, or a side salad.

Creamy Broccoli and Leek Soup

VEGETARIAN, GLUTEN FREE, DAIRY FREE
PREP TIME: 10 MIN **COOK TIME:** 20 MIN **SERVINGS:** 4
Calories: 100, Carbs: 10g, Fat: 3g, Protein: 3g, Fiber: 3g, Sodium: 320mg

- 2 cups broccoli florets
- 1 medium leek, thinly sliced
- 2 garlic cloves, minced
- 1 medium potato, peeled and diced
- 3 cups vegetable broth
- 1 tbsp olive oil
- ½ cup coconut milk (unsweetened)
- ¼ tsp smoked paprika
- Salt and pepper, to taste

1. In a large pot, heat olive oil over medium heat. Sauté the garlic and leek for about 5 minutes until softened.
2. Add the broccoli, diced potato, and vegetable broth to the pot. Bring to a boil, then reduce the heat and simmer for 15 minutes until the vegetables are tender.
3. Puree the soup using an immersion blender or a standard blender until smooth. Stir in the coconut milk and smoked paprika.
4. Season with salt and pepper to taste. Serve warm, garnished with a sprinkle of smoked paprika or fresh herbs.

Zucchini & Basil Bliss Soup

VEGETARIAN, GLUTEN FREE, DAIRY FREE
PREP TIME: 10 MIN **COOK TIME:** 15 MIN **SERVINGS:** 4
Calories: 95, Carbs: 12g, Fat: 4g, Protein: 3g, Fiber: 3g, Sodium: 300mg

- 3 medium zucchinis, sliced
- 1 medium onion, diced
- 2 cups vegetable broth
- 1 tbsp olive oil
- 8-10 fresh basil leaves
- 1 clove garlic, minced
- ½ cup coconut milk
- ¼ cup nutritional yeast

1. In a pot, heat the olive oil over medium heat. The chopped onion should be tender and transparent after 5 minutes of sautéing.
2. Sauté the zucchini slices and minced garlic for a further five minutes.
3. Bring to a boil after adding the vegetable broth. Simmer for ten minutes on low heat.
4. Add the coconut milk and nutritional yeast to the soup after blending it until it's smooth.
5. Add the fresh basil leaves and gently mix to blend before serving.

Spicy Beetroot and Ginger Delight Soup

VEGETARIAN, GLUTEN FREE, DAIRY FREE
PREP TIME: 10 MIN **COOK TIME:** 15 MIN **SERVINGS:** 4
Calories: 120, Carbs: 16g, Fat: 5g, Protein: 2g, Fiber: 3g, Sodium: 300mg

- 3 medium beetroots, peeled and chopped
- 1 tbsp grated ginger
- 2 cups vegetable broth
- 1 tbsp olive oil
- 1 pinch ground coriander
- ½ medium onion, diced
- ½ cup coconut milk
- 1 tbsp fresh lime juice

1. Heat olive oil in a large pot over medium heat.
2. Add the diced onion, ground coriander, and grated ginger. Sauté for 2–3 minutes until fragrant.
3. Add the chopped beetroots and cook for 2–3 minutes, stirring occasionally.
4. Pour in the vegetable broth and bring to a boil. Reduce heat and simmer for 15–20 minutes, or until the beetroots are tender.
5. Remove from heat and carefully puree the soup with an immersion blender or in a standard blender until smooth.
6. Stir in the coconut milk and lime juice. Adjust seasoning as needed and serve warm.

Creamy Potato Leek Soup

VEGETARIAN, GLUTEN FREE, DAIRY FREE
PREP TIME: 10 MIN **COOK TIME:** 20 MIN **SERVINGS:** 4
Calories: 145, Carbs: 25g, Fat: 4g, Protein: 3g, Fiber: 3g, Sodium: 310mg

- 3 medium potatoes, peeled and diced
- 1 medium leek, thinly sliced
- 2 cups vegetable broth
- 1 tbsp olive oil
- 1 pinch thyme
- ½ cup unsweetened almond milk
- ½ tsp garlic powder
- Salt and pepper, to taste

1. Heat the olive oil in a saucepan over medium heat.

For five minutes, sauté the leek slices until they are soft.

2. Add the diced potatoes and veggie broth. After bringing to a boil, simmer for 15 minutes or until the potatoes are tender.
3. Blend the soup until it's smooth. Add the garlic powder, salt, pepper, and unsweetened almond milk and stir. Before serving, warm up and add the thyme.

Smoky Chicken and Butternut Squash Soup

GLUTEN FREE, DAIRY FREE
PREP TIME: 05 MIN **COOK TIME:** 20 MIN **SERVINGS:** 4
Calories: 160, Carbs: 18g, Fat: 4g, Protein: 14g, Fiber: 3g, Sodium: 300mg

- 200g cooked chicken breast, shredded
- 2 cups butternut squash, peeled and diced
- 1 medium onion, diced
- 2 cups chicken broth
- 1 tbsp olive oil
- 1 pinch smoked paprika
- ½ tsp garlic powder
- ¼ tsp ground cumin
- Salt and pepper, to taste
- 1 tbsp fresh parsley (optional for garnish)

1. Heat the olive oil in a saucepan over medium heat. Sauté the diced onion for 3–5 minutes until tender.
2. Add the diced butternut squash, garlic powder, smoked paprika, and cumin. Cook for 2 minutes, stirring occasionally.
3. Pour in the chicken broth and bring to a boil. Reduce the heat and simmer for 15 minutes, or until the butternut squash is tender.
4. Use an immersion blender to puree the soup until smooth, leaving some texture if desired.
5. Stir in the shredded chicken and cook for an additional 2–3 minutes to heat through.
6. Season with salt and pepper. Garnish with fresh parsley if desired and serve warm.

Turmeric Lemon Chickpea Soup

VEGETARIAN, GLUTEN FREE, DAIRY FREE
PREP TIME: 05 MIN **COOK TIME:** 15 MIN **SERVINGS:** 4
Calories: 140, Carbs: 22g, Fat: 4g, Protein: 6g, Fiber: 5g, Sodium: 290mg

- 1 can (15 oz) chickpeas, rinsed and drained
- 3 cups vegetable broth
- 2 tbsp fresh lemon juice
- 1 tbsp olive oil
- 1 pinch ground turmeric
- 1 medium carrot, peeled and diced
- 1 small celery stalk, diced
- ½ tsp cumin powder

1. Heat the olive oil in a saucepan over medium heat. For two to three minutes, sauté the celery, carrot, and chickpeas.
2. Add the cumin powder and ground turmeric, and simmer for one minute.
3. Bring to a boil after adding the vegetable broth. Simmer for ten minutes on low heat.
4. Before serving, stir in the fresh lemon juice.

Velvety Parsnip and Apple Soup

VEGETARIAN, GLUTEN FREE, DAIRY FREE
PREP TIME: 05 MIN **COOK TIME:** 15 MIN **SERVINGS:** 4
Calories: 130, Carbs: 22g, Fat: 3g, Protein: 2g, Fiber: 5g, Sodium: 300mg

- 3 medium parsnips, peeled and diced
- 1 medium onion, diced
- 2 cups vegetable broth
- 1 tbsp olive oil
- 1 pinch nutmeg
- 1 medium apple, peeled and diced
- ½ tsp ground ginger

1. In a pot, heat the olive oil over medium heat. Sauté the diced onion for 5 minutes, until soft.
2. Add the diced parsnips and cook for 5 minutes.
3. Add the diced apple, vegetable broth, and bring to a boil. Simmer until the parsnips are soft, about 15 minutes.
4. Stir in the nutmeg and ground ginger. Blend the soup until smooth and serve warm.

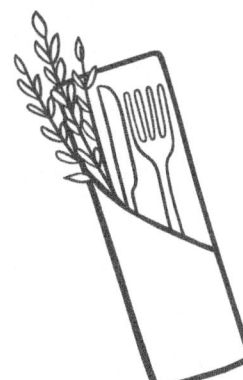

Cod and Potato Chowder

GLUTEN FREE, DAIRY FREE
PREP TIME: 10 MIN **COOK TIME:** 20 MIN **SERVINGS:** 4
Calories: 240, Carbs: 22g, Fat: 8g, Protein: 22g, Fiber: 3g, Sodium: 290mg

- ½ lb cod fillet, cut into chunks
- 2 small potatoes, diced
- 2 medium carrots, peeled and sliced
- 3 cups vegetable broth
- 1 cup almond milk (or any dairy-free milk)
- 1 tbsp olive oil
- 1 pinch smoked paprika

1. Heat the olive oil in a large pot over medium heat. Sauté the diced potatoes and carrots for about 5 minutes, stirring occasionally.
2. Add the vegetable broth to the pot and bring to a simmer. Cook for 8-10 minutes, or until the potatoes are tender.
3. Stir in the almond milk and smoked paprika, then add the cod fillet chunks. Simmer for another 5-7 minutes, or until the cod is fully cooked and flakes easily with a fork.
4. Taste and adjust seasoning as needed.
5. Serve warm, optionally garnished with fresh herbs like parsley or dill for extra flavor.

Herb Beef Soup

GLUTEN FREE, DAIRY FREE
PREP TIME: 05 MIN **COOK TIME:** 15 MIN **SERVINGS:** 4
Calories: 220, Carbs: 7g, Fat: 14g, Protein: 20g, Fiber: 3g, Sodium: 350mg

- ½ lb ground beef
- 3 cups beef broth
- ½ cup diced green beans
- ½ cup diced tomatoes
- 1 tbsp olive oil
- 1 pinch dried rosemary
- ¼ cup chopped kale

1. In a pot, brown the ground beef over medium heat. Remove extra fat.
2. Add the beef broth, green beans, diced tomatoes, and chopped kale. Stir to combine.
3. Simmer for 10 minutes, allowing the vegetables to soften.
4. Serve hot after adding rosemary.

Creamy Pea and Sweet Potato Soup

VEGETARIAN, GLUTEN FREE, DAIRY FREE
PREP TIME: 05 MIN **COOK TIME:** 15 MIN **SERVINGS:** 4
Calories: 130, Carbs: 22g, Fat: 3g, Protein: 5g, Fiber: 5g, Sodium: 270mg

- 2 cups frozen peas
- 1 medium leek, sliced
- 2 cups vegetable broth
- 1 tbsp olive oil
- 1 pinch black pepper
- 2 medium sweet potatoes, peeled and diced
- ½ cup fresh mint leaves

1. In a pot, heat the olive oil over medium heat. Sauté the sliced leek for about 5 minutes until tender.
2. Add the diced sweet potatoes and cook for another 2 minutes.
3. Pour in the vegetable broth and frozen peas. Bring to a boil, then simmer for 10 minutes or until the potatoes are soft.
4. Add black pepper to taste and stir in the fresh mint leaves. Blend until smooth and serve warm.

Roasted Butternut Squash and Cauliflower Soup

VEGETARIAN, GLUTEN FREE, DAIRY FREE
PREP TIME: 05 MIN **COOK TIME:** 20 MIN **SERVINGS:** 4
Calories: 140, Carbs: 25g, Fat: 3g, Protein: 5g, Fiber: 4g, Sodium: 230mg

- 2 cups butternut squash, peeled and cubed
- 2 cups cauliflower florets
- 1 medium onion, diced
- 3 cups vegetable broth
- 1 tbsp olive oil
- 1 tsp ground cumin
- ½ tsp turmeric
- ¼ tsp ground cinnamon
- Salt and pepper, to taste
- ¼ cup coconut milk (optional for extra creaminess)

1. Preheat your oven to 400°F (200°C). Toss the butternut squash and cauliflower with olive oil, salt, and pepper. Spread them out on a baking sheet and roast for 20 minutes or until tender.
2. In a large pot, sauté the diced onion for 5 minutes until softened.
3. Add the roasted squash and cauliflower to the pot along with vegetable broth, cumin, turmeric, and cinnamon. Bring to a boil, then simmer for 10 minutes.

4. Use an immersion blender to puree the soup until smooth, or transfer to a blender.
5. Stir in coconut milk, adjust seasonings, and serve warm.

Lemon Chicken and Vegetable Orzo Soup

GLUTEN FREE, DAIRY FREE
PREP TIME: 05 MIN **COOK TIME:** 15 MIN **SERVINGS:** 4
Calories: 180, Carbs: 22g, Fat: 4g, Protein: 15g, Fiber: 3g, Sodium: 380mg

- 1 cup shredded cooked chicken
- 3 cups chicken broth
- ½ cup cooked orzo
- 2 tbsp fresh lemon juice
- 1 tsp olive oil
- 1 medium carrot, diced
- 1 small zucchini, diced

1. In a pot, warm the chicken broth over medium heat.
2. Add the cooked orzo, shredded chicken, diced carrot, and zucchini to the broth. Simmer for about 5 minutes until the vegetables are tender.
3. Add the fresh lemon juice and olive oil. Stir well, and serve warm.

Spicy Shrimp and Fennel Citrus Soup

GLUTEN FREE, DAIRY FREE
PREP TIME: 05 MIN **COOK TIME:** 15 MIN **SERVINGS:** 4
Calories: 140, Carbs: 6g, Fat: 4g, Protein: 18g, Fiber: 2g, Sodium: 290mg

- ½ lb. shrimp, peeled and deveined
- 1 small fennel bulb, thinly sliced
- 3 cups fish or vegetable broth
- 1 tbsp olive oil
- 1 pinch red pepper flakes
- 1 medium orange, juiced and zested
- 1 small carrot, diced

1. Heat the olive oil in a big pot over medium heat.
2. Cook for 5 minutes, stirring periodically, until the carrot and thinly sliced fennel are tender.
3. Add the vegetable or fish broth and bring to a low boil. Lower the heat until it simmers.
4. Pour the orange juice, zest, red pepper flakes, and shrimp into the pot. Simmer until the shrimp are pink and cooked through, 3 to 5 minutes.
5. Serve the soup hot after ladling it into dishes.

Hearty Turkey Meatball and Kale Soup

GLUTEN FREE, DAIRY FREE
PREP TIME: 10 MIN **COOK TIME:** 20 MIN **SERVINGS:** 4
Calories: 180, Carbs: 6g, Fat: 7g, Protein: 23g, Fiber: 2g, Sodium: 320mg

- 12 small turkey meatballs (store-bought or homemade)
- 3 cups chicken broth
- 1 cup baby kale or arugula
- 1 tsp olive oil
- 1 pinch dried oregano
- ½ cup diced carrots
- 1 small zucchini, sliced

1. In a pot, heat the olive oil over medium heat. Cook the turkey meatballs for approximately five minutes, or until they are gently browned.
2. Add the chicken broth, bringing it to a boil. Simmer for ten minutes on low heat.
3. Add the oregano, diced carrots, zucchini, and baby kale, stirring to combine. Cook for an additional 2 minutes.
4. Serve warm and enjoy!

Spinach-Chickpea Comfort Soup

VEGETARIAN, GLUTEN FREE, DAIRY FREE
PREP TIME: 05 MIN **COOK TIME:** 15 MIN **SERVINGS:** 4
Calories: 170, Carbs: 22g, Fat: 5g, Protein: 7g, Fiber: 7g, Sodium: 280mg

- 1 can (15 oz) chickpeas, drained and rinsed
- 3 cups vegetable broth
- 2 tbsp fresh lemon juice
- 1 tbsp olive oil
- 1 pinch ground cumin
- 2 cups fresh spinach, chopped
- 1 small carrot, diced

1. In a pot, heat the olive oil over medium heat. Sauté the chickpeas for two minutes.
2. Add the diced carrot and cook for another two minutes.
3. Add the vegetable broth and bring to a simmer. Cook for about ten minutes.
4. Stir in cumin, fresh lemon juice, and chopped spinach. Let it cook for an additional 2-3 minutes until the spinach wilts.
5. You can leave the soup chunky or partially blend it for a creamy texture. Warm up and serve.

Zucchini-Infused Chicken Soup

GLUTEN FREE, DAIRY FREE
PREP TIME: 05 MIN **COOK TIME:** 20 MIN **SERVINGS:** 4
Calories: 150, Carbs: 12g, Fat: 4g, Protein: 14g, Fiber: 2g, Sodium: 300mg

- **1 cup shredded cooked chicken**
- **3 cups chicken broth**
- **½ cup diced carrots**
- **½ cup diced zucchini**
- **1 small potato, diced**
- **2 garlic cloves, minced**
- **1 tbsp olive oil**
- **¼ tsp smoked paprika**
- **½ tsp dried thyme**
- **1 tbsp fresh parsley, chopped (for garnish)**
- **Salt and pepper, to taste**

1. Heat olive oil in a large pot over medium heat. Sauté the minced garlic for 1–2 minutes until fragrant.
2. Add the diced carrots, zucchini, and potato, and cook for 5 minutes, stirring occasionally.
3. Stir in the chicken broth, smoked paprika, and thyme. Bring to a boil, then reduce heat to a simmer. Cook for 10–12 minutes or until the vegetables are tender.
4. Add the shredded chicken, stir, and simmer for 3–5 minutes to heat through. Season with salt and pepper to taste.
5. Serve warm, garnished with freshly chopped parsley.

Ocean Kissed Tomato Soup with Sea Bass

GLUTEN FREE, DAIRY FREE
PREP TIME: 05 MIN **COOK TIME:** 20 MIN **SERVINGS:** 4
Calories: 130, Carbs: 6g, Fat: 4g, Protein: 19g, Fiber: 2g, Sodium: 350mg

- **½ lb sea bass fillets, diced**
- **3 cups fish broth or water**
- **½ cup diced tomatoes**
- **½ cup diced cucumber**
- **¼ cup kalamata olives, sliced**
- **1 tbsp olive oil**
- **1 pinch dried basil**

1. In a medium pot, heat olive oil over medium heat.
2. Add the diced tomatoes and cook for 3-4 minutes, allowing them to soften and release their juices.
3. Pour in the fish broth or water, then bring to a gentle boil.
4. Add the diced sea bass, diced cucumber, sliced olives, and dried basil. Reduce heat to a simmer and cook for 8-10 minutes, or until the fish is fully cooked and flakes easily.
5. Ladle the soup into bowls and serve hot.

Spiced Lamb and Vegetable Soup

GLUTEN FREE, DAIRY FREE
PREP TIME: 05 MIN **COOK TIME:** 20 MIN **SERVINGS:** 4
Calories: 190, Carbs: 10g, Fat: 10g, Protein: 17g, Fiber: 3g, Sodium: 240mg

- **½ lb ground lamb**
- **3 cups beef or lamb broth**
- **½ cup diced zucchini**
- **½ cup diced carrots**
- **½ cup diced sweet potato**
- **1 pinch ground cumin**

1. Brown the ground lamb in a saucepan over medium heat. Remove extra fat.
2. Add the broth, chopped carrots, zucchini, and sweet potato. Simmer for 15 minutes until vegetables are tender.
3. Before serving, stir in the cumin.

Minestrone Soup

VEGETARIAN, GLUTEN FREE, DAIRY FREE
PREP TIME: 05 MIN **COOK TIME:** 25 MIN **SERVINGS:** 4
Calories: 110, Carbs: 18g, Fat: 1g, Protein: 6g, Fiber: 5g, Sodium: 250mg

- **1 cup canned diced tomatoes**
- **1 cup vegetable broth**
- **1 cup zucchini, diced**
- **1 cup canned cannellini beans, rinsed and drained**
- **½ tsp dried Italian seasoning**

1. Heat a medium-sized pot over medium heat. Add the diced tomatoes, vegetable broth, and Italian seasoning. Stir to combine and bring the mixture to a boil.
2. Reduce the heat to low, add the diced zucchini, and let it simmer for 10 minutes, stirring occasionally.
3. Add the cannellini beans to the pot and cook for an additional 5 minutes.
4. Remove from heat and serve the soup warm.

Creamy Salmon Soup

GLUTEN FREE, DAIRY FREE
PREP TIME: 05 MIN **COOK TIME:** 15 MIN **SERVINGS:** 4
Calories: 250 Carbs: 10g Fat: 12g Protein: 22g
Fiber: 3g Sodium: 450mg

- 300g fresh salmon fillet, skin removed and cut into cubes
- 1 medium potato, peeled and diced
- 2 medium carrots, peeled and sliced
- 4 cups vegetable broth (or fish broth)
- 1 cup coconut milk
- 1 tbsp fresh dill, chopped
- 1 tsp garlic powder
- ½ tsp salt
- ¼ tsp black pepper
- 1 tbsp lemon juice

1. In a large pot, bring the vegetable broth to a boil. Add the diced potato and sliced carrots. Reduce heat and simmer for 10-12 minutes, until the vegetables are tender.
2. Add the cubed salmon to the pot and cook for 4-5 minutes, until the salmon is fully cooked and flakes easily.
3. Pour in the coconut milk and stir to combine.
4. Add the fresh dill, garlic powder, salt, black pepper, and lemon juice. Stir well and simmer for an additional 2-3 minutes.
5. Taste and adjust seasoning if needed, and serve hot.

YOUR FREE BONUSES!

To help you ease into the Mediterranean Diet, I've created two bonus books specially designed to enhance your skill sets in cooking and food preparation so that you can optimize your health with greater ease.

- **Meal Prep and Food Repurposing Guide** where you'll find *practical tips* for saving money, repurposing ingredients, and minimizing food waste. From pantry stocking tips to batch cooking and quick meal formulae, you'll be equipped to plan, prep and cook your meals in a more efficient way.

- **A Reference Book of 70 Classic Mediterranean Recipes with Full Colored Pictures** where a collection of signature dishes comes alive with *vibrant, full-colored photos* forming a foundational compass so you can identify the key elements that make up a dish in a food category. Making you more confident in creating delectable Mediterranean dishes.

Get access to the bonus ebooks by copying the below link and pasting it in your browser or scanning the QR code with your mobile phone's camera.

https://heartbookspress.com/SuperEasyMediterranean-FreeBonuses

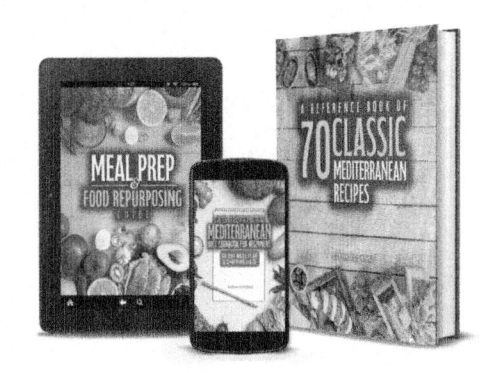

CHAPTER 6
SALADS

A symphony of colors, flavors, and textures, salads are the cornerstone of Mediterranean cuisine. This chapter explores a variety of refreshing and nourishing salads, from simple green salads to hearty grain bowls.

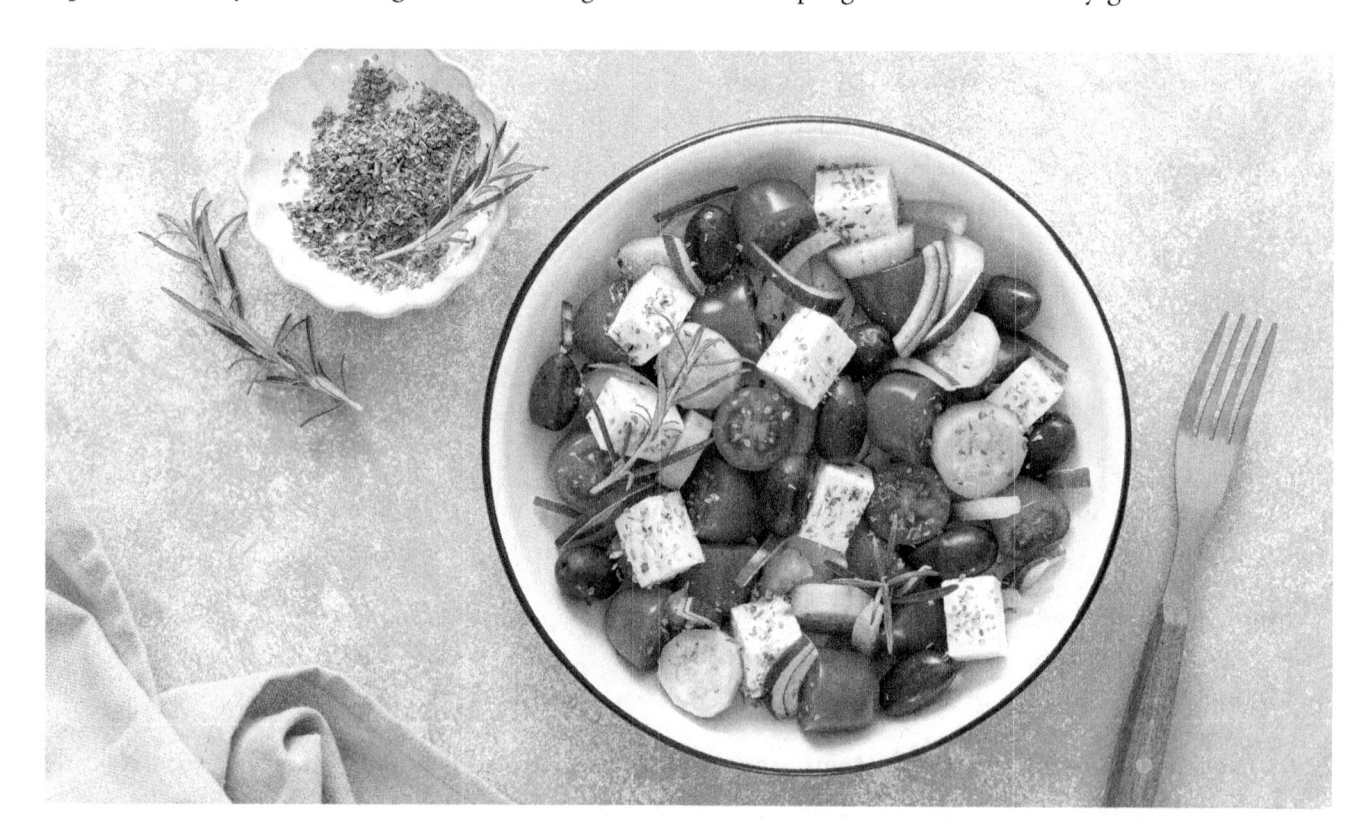

TIPS:

- Add a protein source, such as grilled chicken, roasted chickpeas, or tofu, to make your salad more filling.

- Combine grains like quinoa, rice, or farro with vegetables, protein, and a flavorful dressing for a hearty and satisfying meal.

- Use leftover grilled vegetables, roasted chicken, or cooked grains to create quick and easy salads.

Simple Greek Salad with Lemon-Olive Dressing

VEGETARIAN, GLUTEN FREE, DAIRY FREE
PREP TIME: 10 MIN **COOK TIME:** 00 MIN **SERVINGS:** 2
Calories: 150, Carbs: 8g, Fat: 11g, Protein: 2g, Fiber: 6g, Sodium: 35mg

- 1 cup diced cucumber
- ½ cup cherry tomatoes, halved
- ¼ cup kalamata olives
- ¼ cup diced red bell pepper
- 1 tsp dried oregano
- ¼ cup diced ripe avocado
- 1 tbsp lemon juice
- 1 tsp olive oil
- ½ tsp Dijon mustard (optional for extra flavor)
- Salt and pepper, to taste

1. In a bowl, combine the cucumber, cherry tomatoes, red bell pepper, avocado, and olives.
2. Sprinkle with dried oregano.
3. In a small bowl, whisk together the lemon juice, olive oil, Dijon mustard (if using), salt, and pepper.
4. Drizzle the dressing over the salad and toss gently to combine.

Grilled Zucchini and Tomato Salad with Lemon Herb Dressing

VEGETARIAN, GLUTEN FREE, DAIRY FREE
PREP TIME: 05 MIN **COOK TIME:** 10 MIN **SERVINGS:** 2
Calories: 120, Carbs: 9g, Fat: 8g, Protein: 2g, Fiber: 3g, Sodium: 15mg

- 2 medium zucchinis, sliced
- 1 tbsp olive oil
- 1 tsp lemon zest
- 1 tsp fresh dill, chopped
- 1 pinch salt
- ¼ cup cherry tomatoes, halved
- 1 tbsp balsamic vinegar
- 1 tbsp fresh basil, chopped

1. Grill zucchini slices for about 5 minutes on each side, until they are soft and faintly browned.
2. Place the grilled zucchini in a bowl and drizzle with olive oil.
3. Add salt, dill, lemon zest, and toss gently to combine.
4. Add halved cherry tomatoes, balsamic vinegar, and fresh basil just before serving.
5. Toss lightly and serve right away.

Zesty Quinoa Power Salad

VEGETARIAN, GLUTEN FREE, DAIRY FREE
PREP TIME: 10 MIN **COOK TIME:** 00 MIN **SERVINGS:** 2
Calories: 230, Carbs: 27g, Fat: 9g, Protein: 6g, Fiber: 6g, Sodium: 25mg

- 1 cup cooked quinoa
- ½ orange, segmented
- ½ cup diced cucumber
- ¼ cup pomegranate seeds
- 2 tbsp chopped almonds
- 1 tbsp lemon juice
- 1 tbsp olive oil
- 1 tsp chopped parsley

1. In a large bowl, combine the cooked quinoa, orange segments, cucumber, pomegranate seeds, and almonds.
2. Drizzle with lemon juice and olive oil.
3. Sprinkle with parsley and gently toss to mix.

Grilled Chicken with Mixed Greens in Creamy Herb Dressing

GLUTEN FREE, DAIRY FREE
PREP TIME: 10 MIN **COOK TIME:** 10 MIN **SERVINGS:** 2
Calories: 270, Carbs: 9g, Fat: 18g, Protein: 23g, Fiber: 3g, Sodium: 120mg

- 1 grilled chicken breast, diced
- ½ cup cherry tomatoes, halved
- 2 cups mixed greens
- ½ cucumber, diced
- ¼ cup red onion, thinly sliced

Creamy Herb Dressing:
- 2 tbsp tahini (or almond butter for a nutty flavor)
- 1 tbsp lemon juice
- 1 tbsp olive oil
- 1 tsp Dijon mustard
- ½ tsp dried dill (or fresh dill, chopped)
- 1 garlic clove, minced
- Salt and pepper, to taste
- 1-2 tbsp water to thin (if needed)

1. Add the chopped chicken, red onion, cucumber, mixed greens, and cherry tomatoes to a big bowl.
2. Mix the tahini, lemon juice, olive oil, Dijon mustard, dill, minced garlic, salt, and pepper in a small bowl. Add water a bit at a time until the dressing achieves the consistency you want if it's too thick.
3. Gently toss the salad after drizzling it with the creamy herb dressing. Serve right away.

Lemon Kissed Grilled Chicken Salad

GLUTEN FREE, DAIRY FREE
PREP TIME: 10 MIN **COOK TIME:** 10 MIN **SERVINGS:** 2
Calories: 270, Carbs: 8g, Fat: 17g, Protein: 23g, Fiber: 4g, Sodium: 75mg

- 1 grilled chicken breast, sliced
- 2 cups mixed greens
- ½ avocado, sliced
- ¼ cup cucumber, sliced
- 1 tbsp red onion, thinly sliced

Dressing:
- 1 tbsp apple cider vinegar
- 1 tsp Dijon mustard
- Salt and pepper, to taste
- 1 tbsp olive oil
- 1 tbsp lemon juice

1. In a bowl, combine the mixed greens, cucumber, and red onion.
2. Place the sliced grilled chicken and avocado on top.
3. In a small bowl, whisk together the olive oil, lemon juice, apple cider vinegar, Dijon mustard, salt, and pepper to make the dressing.
4. Pour the dressing over the salad and toss gently.
5. Serve right away.

Grilled Steak Salad with Balsamic Vinaigrette

GLUTEN FREE, DAIRY FREE
PREP TIME: 10 MIN **COOK TIME:** 10 MIN **SERVINGS:** 2
Calories: 265, Carbs: 6g, Fat: 17g, Protein: 22g, Fiber: 3g, Sodium: 70mg

- 1 grilled steak (4 oz), sliced
- 2 cups romaine lettuce
- ½ red bell pepper, sliced
- ¼ cup cucumber, diced
- ¼ cup cherry tomatoes, halved

Balsamic Vinaigrette:
- 1 tbsp balsamic vinegar
- 2 tbsp olive oil
- 1 tsp Dijon mustard
- 1 tsp honey (optional)
- Salt and pepper, to taste

1. In a salad bowl, arrange the romaine lettuce, red bell pepper, cucumber, and cherry tomatoes.
2. Place the sliced grilled steak on top.
3. In a small bowl, whisk together the balsamic vinegar, olive oil, Dijon mustard, and honey. Add salt and pepper to taste.
4. Drizzle the balsamic vinaigrette over the salad and toss lightly before serving.

Fattoush Salad

VEGETARIAN, GLUTEN FREE, DAIRY FREE
PREP TIME: 10 MIN **COOK TIME:** 00 MIN **SERVINGS:** 4
Calories: 70, Carbs: 3g, Fat: 6g, Protein: 1g, Fiber: 1g, Sodium: 5mg

- 1 cup lettuce, chopped
- 1 cup cucumbers, diced
- ½ cup cherry tomatoes, halved
- 2 tbsp olive oil
- 1 tbsp lemon juice

1. In a large salad bowl, combine the lettuce, cucumbers, and cherry tomatoes.
2. In a small bowl, whisk together the olive oil and lemon juice to create a simple dressing.
3. Drizzle the dressing over the salad and toss gently to coat all the vegetables evenly. Serve immediately.

Grilled Chicken and Roasted Bell Pepper Salad with Tahini-Garlic Dressing

GLUTEN FREE, DAIRY FREE
PREP TIME: 10 MIN **COOK TIME:** 10 MIN **SERVINGS:** 2
Calories: 260, Carbs: 10g, Fat: 15g, Protein: 22g, Fiber: 3g, Sodium: 90mg

- 1 grilled chicken breast, sliced
- 1 cup roasted red bell pepper strips (jarred or homemade)
- 2 cups mixed greens
- ¼ cucumber, thinly sliced
- ¼ red onion, thinly sliced

Tahini-Garlic Dressing:
- 2 tbsp tahini
- 1 tbsp apple cider vinegar
- 1 tsp maple syrup (optional)
- 1 small garlic clove, minced
- 2 tbsp water (to thin, if needed)
- Salt and pepper, to taste

1. Arrange the sliced grilled chicken, roasted red bell peppers, cucumber, and red onion over a bed of mixed greens.
2. In a small bowl, whisk together the tahini, apple cider vinegar, maple syrup (if using), minced garlic, and water until smooth. Add salt and pepper to taste. Adjust the thickness of the dressing by adding more water if necessary.
3. Drizzle the tahini-garlic dressing over the salad and toss gently to coat. Serve immediately.

Garden Fresh Watermelon-Cucumber Salad

VEGETARIAN, GLUTEN FREE

PREP TIME: 10 MIN **COOK TIME:** 00 MIN **SERVINGS:** 2

Calories: 170, Carbs: 14g, Fat: 10g, Protein: 5g, Fiber: 2g, Sodium: 140mg

- 1 cup diced watermelon
- ½ cup cucumber, diced
- ¼ cup crumbled feta cheese
- 2 tbsp red onion, thinly sliced
- 1 tbsp toasted sunflower seeds
- 1 tbsp olive oil
- 1 tsp fresh mint, chopped
- 1 pinch black pepper

1. Put the feta cheese, red onion, cucumber, and watermelon in a bowl.
2. Sprinkle the sunflower seeds on top for crunch.
3. Add a little olive oil and season with black pepper and mint.
4. Toss gently to mix, then serve right away.

Tuna and White Bean Salad with Creamy Mustard Dressing

GLUTEN FREE, DAIRY FREE

PREP TIME: 10 MIN **COOK TIME:** 00 MIN **SERVINGS:** 2

Calories: 250, Carbs: 15g, Fat: 12g, Protein: 26g, Fiber: 6g, Sodium: 180mg

- 1 can (5 oz) tuna in water, drained
- ½ cup white beans, rinsed
- ¼ cup diced cucumber
- ¼ cup cherry tomatoes, halved
- ¼ cup red onion, thinly sliced

Dressing:
- 1 tbsp olive oil
- 1 tbsp Dijon mustard
- 1 tbsp red wine vinegar
- 1 tsp lemon juice
- ½ tsp honey (optional)
- Salt and pepper, to taste

1. In a bowl, combine the tuna, white beans, cucumber, tomatoes, and red onion.
2. In a separate bowl, whisk together the olive oil, Dijon mustard, red wine vinegar, lemon juice, and honey (if using). Season with salt and pepper to taste.
3. Pour the dressing over the salad and toss gently to combine.
4. Before serving, sprinkle chopped parsley on top.

Roasted Carrot And Arugula Salad with Dijon Vinaigrette

VEGETARIAN, GLUTEN FREE, DAIRY FREE

PREP TIME: 10 MIN **COOK TIME:** 10 MIN **SERVINGS:** 2

Calories: 230, Carbs: 26g, Fat: 8g, Protein: 8g, Fiber: 7g, Sodium: 50mg

- 1 cup cooked green lentils
- 2 medium carrots, roasted and sliced
- 2 cups arugula
- ¼ cup red onion, thinly sliced
- ½ cup cucumber, sliced

Dijon Vinaigrette:
- 1 tbsp Dijon mustard
- 1 tbsp red wine vinegar
- 1 tbsp olive oil
- 1 tsp honey or maple syrup (optional)
- Salt and pepper, to taste

1. Preheat the oven to 400°F (200°C).
2. Toss the sliced carrots with olive oil and a pinch of salt (optional). Spread evenly on a baking sheet and roast for 20 minutes, turning halfway through, until tender and lightly caramelized.
3. In a bowl, combine the roasted carrots, arugula, cooked lentils, red onion, and cucumber.
4. In a small bowl, whisk together Dijon mustard, red wine vinegar, olive oil, honey/maple syrup (if using), salt, and pepper until smooth.
5. Drizzle the Dijon vinaigrette over the salad and toss gently before serving.

Mediterranean-Inspired Lentil Parsley Salad

VEGETARIAN, GLUTEN FREE, DAIRY FREE

PREP TIME: 10 MIN **COOK TIME:** 00 MIN **SERVINGS:** 2

Calories: 220, Carbs: 25g, Fat: 9g, Protein: 10g, Fiber: 9g, Sodium: 190mg

- 1 cup cooked green lentils
- ½ cup diced cucumber
- 1 tbsp olive oil
- 1 tbsp lemon juice
- 1 tsp chopped fresh parsley
- ¼ cup cherry tomatoes, halved
- ¼ cup Kalamata olives, pitted and sliced
- 1 tbsp red onion, finely chopped

1. In a bowl, combine the cooked lentils, cucumber, cherry tomatoes, olives, red onion, and parsley.
2. Drizzle with olive oil and lemon juice.
3. Gently toss and serve cold.

Grilled Mediterranean Salmon Salad with Avocado Dressing

GLUTEN FREE, DAIRY FREE
PREP TIME: 10 MIN **COOK TIME:** 10 MIN **SERVINGS:** 2
Calories: 260, Carbs: 7g, Fat: 18g, Protein: 26g, Fiber: 5g, Sodium: 180mg

- 1 grilled salmon fillet, flaked
- 2 cups baby spinach
- ¼ cup cucumber, diced
- ¼ cup cherry tomatoes, halved

Avocado Dressing:
- ½ avocado
- 1 tbsp olive oil
- 1 tbsp apple cider vinegar
- 1 tsp Dijon mustard
- 1 tbsp water (to adjust consistency)
- Salt and pepper, to taste

1. In a bowl, arrange the baby spinach as the base.
2. Add the flaked salmon, cucumber, and cherry tomatoes on top of the spinach.
3. In a blender, combine the avocado, olive oil, apple cider vinegar, Dijon mustard, and water. Blend until smooth.
4. Drizzle the avocado dressing over the salad and toss lightly before serving.

Roasted Cauliflower and Chickpea Salad with Lemon-Tahini Dressing

VEGETARIAN, GLUTEN FREE, DAIRY FREE
PREP TIME: 10 MIN **COOK TIME:** 20 MIN **SERVINGS:** 2
Calories: 280, Carbs: 32g, Fat: 14g, Protein: 10g, Fiber: 9g, Sodium: 70mg

- 1 cup cauliflower florets, roasted
- 1 cup chickpeas, roasted
- 2 cups spinach
- ½ red onion, thinly sliced
- ¼ cup pomegranate seeds

Lemon-Tahini Dressing:
- 1 tbsp tahini
- 1 tbsp lemon juice
- 1 tbsp olive oil
- 1 tsp maple syrup (optional for sweetness)
- Salt and pepper, to taste

1. Preheat oven to 400°F (200°C). Toss cauliflower florets and chickpeas with a drizzle of olive oil, season with salt (optional), and roast for 20 minutes, stirring halfway through.
2. In a bowl, combine the roasted cauliflower, roasted chickpeas, spinach, red onion, and pomegranate seeds.
3. In a small bowl, whisk together tahini, lemon juice, olive oil, maple syrup, salt, and pepper until smooth.
4. Drizzle the dressing over the salad and toss gently before serving.

Vibrant Veggie Chickpea Salad

VEGETARIAN, GLUTEN FREE, DAIRY FREE
PREP TIME: 10 MIN **COOK TIME:** 00 MIN **SERVINGS:** 2
Calories: 200, Carbs: 26g, Fat: 8g, Protein: 7g, Fiber: 6g, Sodium: 150mg

- 1 cup canned chickpeas, rinsed and drained
- ½ cup diced cucumber
- ¼ cup diced bell peppers (any color)
- ¼ cup cherry tomatoes, halved
- 1 tbsp chopped fresh parsley
- 1 tbsp lemon juice
- 1 tbsp olive oil
- 1 pinch cumin powder

1. Put the chickpeas, bell peppers, cucumber, cherry tomatoes, and parsley in a bowl.
2. Drizzle the mixture with olive oil and lemon juice.
3. To ensure all ingredients are uniformly coated, add cumin powder and mix gently.
4. For a cool salad, serve chilled.

Tabbouleh

VEGETARIAN, DAIRY FREE
PREP TIME: 10 MIN **COOK TIME:** 00 MIN **SERVINGS:** 4
Calories: 80, Carbs: 9g, Fat: 4g, Protein: 1g, Fiber: 2g, Sodium: 5mg

- 1 cup parsley, finely chopped
- ½ cup cherry tomatoes, diced
- ¼ cup bulgur wheat, soaked in hot water (quinoa for gluten free)
- 2 tbsp lemon juice
- 1 tbsp olive oil

1. Place the soaked bulgur wheat in a large mixing bowl.
2. Add the chopped parsley, diced tomatoes, lemon juice, and olive oil.
3. Toss the mixture well until all ingredients are evenly combined. Serve chilled or at room temperature.

Shrimp and Cucumber Citrus Salad

GLUTEN FREE, DAIRY FREE
PREP TIME: 10 MIN **COOK TIME:** 05 MIN **SERVINGS:** 2
Calories: 240, Carbs: 12g, Fat: 12g, Protein: 22g,
Fiber: 3g, Sodium: 190mg

- 1 cup cooked shrimp, peeled and deveined
- 1 cup orange segments (or diced grapefruit)
- 2 cups mixed greens
- ½ cup diced cucumber
- ¼ cup sliced red onion
- 1 tbsp chopped dill or parsley
- 1 tbsp olive oil
- 1 tbsp lemon juice

1. Put the shrimp, orange segments, mixed greens, cucumber, red onion, and dill in a big bowl.
2. Pour lemon juice and olive oil over it. Toss gently to coat the salad evenly.
3. Serve right away as a side dish or as a light and refreshing supper.

Crunchy Rainbow Salad with Honey-Lime Dressing

VEGETARIAN, GLUTEN FREE, DAIRY FREE
PREP TIME: 10 MIN **COOK TIME:** 00 MIN **SERVINGS:** 2
Calories: 190, Carbs: 17g, Fat: 13g, Protein: 3g, Fiber: 4g, Sodium: 20mg

- 1 cup shredded red cabbage
- ½ cup grated carrots
- ½ cup diced cucumber
- ¼ cup thinly sliced red bell pepper
- ¼ cup chopped fresh parsley
- 2 tbsp roasted sunflower seeds

Dressing:
- 2 tbsp lime juice
- 1 tsp honey (or maple syrup for vegan)
- 1 tbsp olive oil
- ½ tsp Dijon mustard
- Salt and pepper, to taste

1. In a large mixing basin, combine the red bell pepper, red cabbage, carrots, cucumber, and parsley. For crunch, scatter toasted sunflower seeds on top.
2. Emulsify the lime juice, honey, olive oil, Dijon mustard, salt, and pepper in a small bowl by whisking them together.
3. To ensure even coating, drizzle the salad with the dressing and toss thoroughly.

4. Serve right away as a light main course or as a cool side.

Spicy Avocado & Quinoa Corn Salad

VEGETARIAN, GLUTEN FREE, DAIRY FREE
PREP TIME: 10 MIN
COOK TIME: 10 MIN (QUINOA PREPARED AHEAD)
SERVINGS: 2
Calories: 230, Carbs: 26g, Fat: 11g, Protein: 6g, Fiber: 5g, Sodium: 15mg

- 1 cup cooked quinoa
- ½ avocado, diced
- 1 tbsp olive oil
- 1 tbsp lime juice
- 1 pinch chili flakes
- ¼ cup corn kernels (cooked or fresh)
- ¼ cup red bell pepper, diced

1. In a bowl, combine the quinoa, avocado, corn, and red bell pepper.
2. Pour some lime juice and olive oil over it.
3. Serve right away after tossing with chili flakes.

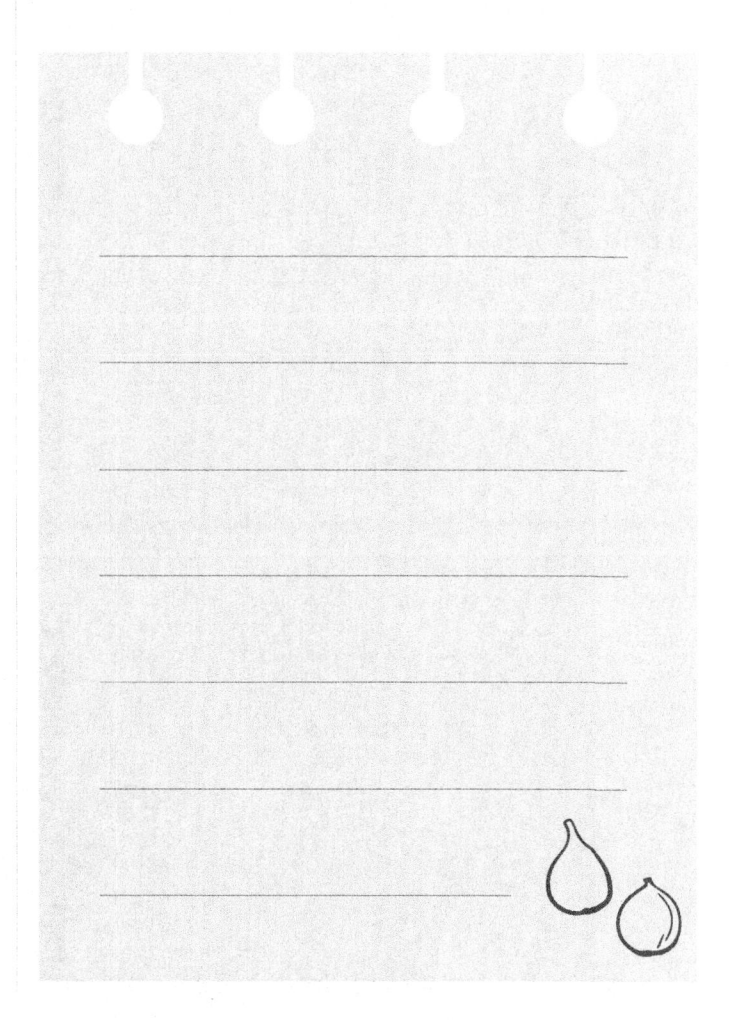

Shrimp and Mango Medley with Cilantro Dressing

GLUTEN FREE, DAIRY FREE
PREP TIME: 10 MIN **COOK TIME:** 05 MIN **SERVINGS:** 2
Calories: 220, Carbs: 15g, Fat: 10g, Protein: 18g, Fiber: 3g, Sodium: 150mg

- 8 shrimp, cooked and peeled
- ½ cup diced mango
- 2 cups arugula
- ¼ cup cucumber, diced
- 1 tbsp red bell pepper, diced

Dressing:
- 1 tbsp olive oil
- 1 tbsp lime juice
- 1 tsp honey
- 1 tbsp fresh cilantro, chopped
- Salt and pepper, to taste

1. Put the red bell pepper, cucumber, arugula, mango, and shrimp in a salad bowl.
2. To make the dressing, combine the olive oil, lime juice, honey, cilantro, salt, and pepper in a small bowl.
3. Drizzle the salad with the dressing and carefully toss.
4. Serve immediately.

Turkey and Pear Salad with Honey Mustard Dressing

GLUTEN FREE, DAIRY FREE
PREP TIME: 10 MIN **COOK TIME:** 00 MIN **SERVINGS:** 2
Calories: 250, Carbs: 16g, Fat: 14g, Protein:

- ½ cup sliced roasted turkey
- 1 pear, thinly sliced
- 2 cups mixed greens
- ¼ cup walnuts, chopped
- ¼ cup crumbled feta (optional)

Honey Mustard Dressing:
- 1 tbsp Dijon mustard
- 1 tbsp honey
- 2 tbsp olive oil
- 1 tsp apple cider vinegar
- Salt and pepper, to taste

1. In a bowl, combine the pear, turkey slices, mixed greens, and walnuts (and feta, if using).
2. In a separate bowl, whisk together Dijon mustard, honey, olive oil, apple cider vinegar, salt, and pepper to create the dressing.
3. Drizzle the honey mustard dressing over the salad and toss gently.
4. Serve right away.

Chickpea and Arugula Salad with Tahini Dressing

VEGETARIAN, GLUTEN FREE, DAIRY FREE
PREP TIME: 10 MIN **COOK TIME:** 00 MIN **SERVINGS:** 2
Calories: 250, Carbs: 30g, Fat: 12g, Protein: 9g, Fiber: 8g, Sodium: 180mg

- 1 cup canned chickpeas, rinsed and drained
- 2 cups arugula
- ½ cucumber, diced
- ¼ cup red onion, thinly sliced
- ½ cup cherry tomatoes, halved

Tahini Dressing:
- 1 tbsp tahini
- 1 tbsp lemon juice
- 1 tbsp water (adjust for consistency)
- 1 tsp olive oil
- 1 garlic clove, minced
- Salt and pepper, to taste

1. In a bowl, combine the arugula, chickpeas, cucumber, red onion, and cherry tomatoes.
2. In a small bowl, whisk together the tahini, lemon juice, water, olive oil, and minced garlic. Adjust with salt and pepper to taste.
3. Pour the tahini dressing over the salad and toss lightly before serving.

CHAPTER 7
VEGETABLES

The Mediterranean diet celebrates the bounty of nature, and vegetables are at its heart. From the vibrant colors of roasted vegetables to the comforting flavors of stewed vegetables, this chapter explores a variety of vegetable dishes that are both delicious and nutritious.

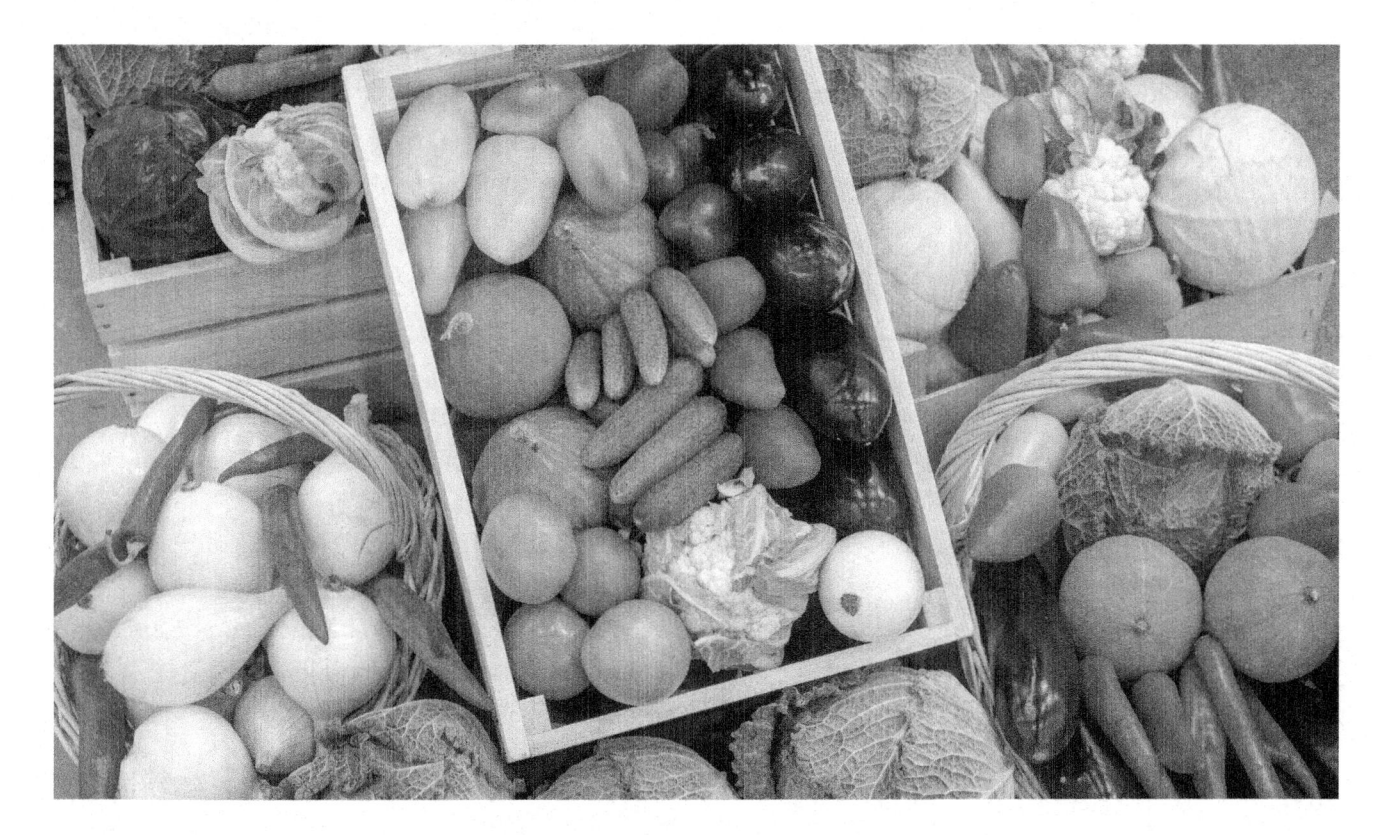

TIPS

- Overcooking vegetables can lead to a mushy texture. Cook them just until tender-crisp.

- Use a variety of colorful vegetables to create visually appealing and nutritious meals.

- Sometimes the simplest preparations are the most delicious. Let the natural flavors of the vegetables shine.

Roasted Zucchini, Squash and Cherry Tomatoes with Red Onion

VEGETARIAN, GLUTEN FREE, DAIRY FREE
PREP TIME: 10 MIN **COOK TIME:** 20 MIN **SERVINGS:** 4
Calories: 85, Carbs: 8g, Fat: 4g, Protein: 2g, Fiber: 3g, Sodium: 10mg

- 2 medium zucchinis, sliced
- 2 medium yellow squash, sliced
- 1 cup cherry tomatoes
- 1 small red onion, thinly sliced
- 1 tbsp olive oil
- 1 tsp garlic powder
- 1 pinch dried thyme

1. Set the oven's temperature to 400°F, or 200°C.
2. Combine the red onion, zucchini, yellow squash, and cherry tomatoes in a large bowl. Sprinkle with dried thyme and garlic powder, drizzle with olive oil, and toss to coat evenly.
3. Arrange the vegetables on a baking sheet in a single layer.
4. The vegetables should be soft and starting to caramelize after 20 minutes of baking in a preheated oven.
5. Take out of the oven and serve hot.

Green Bean Medley with Roasted Garlic and Almond Bliss

VEGETARIAN, GLUTEN FREE, DAIRY FREE
PREP TIME: 05 MIN **COOK TIME:** 12 MIN **SERVINGS:** 4
Calories: 130, Carbs: 13g, Fat: 7g, Protein: 4g, Fiber: 4g, Sodium: 15mg

- 300g green beans, trimmed
- 2 cloves garlic, minced
- 1 cup cherry tomatoes, halved
- ¼ cup sliced almonds
- ½ cup sliced cremini mushrooms
- 1 tbsp fresh lemon juice
- 1 tbsp olive oil
- 1 pinch salt
- 1 pinch black pepper

1. In a large skillet, heat the olive oil over medium heat. Sauté the mushrooms and green beans for five minutes.
2. To the skillet, add the cherry tomatoes and minced garlic. Continue cooking, stirring occasionally, for another 4 to 5 minutes, or until the beans are cooked through, the mushrooms are mushy, and the tomatoes have softened.
3. Add the almond slices and cook for one minute, or until they are just beginning to toast.
4. Take off the heat, add salt and black pepper, then squeeze in some fresh lemon juice. Enjoy warm!

Baked Stuffed Zucchini Boats with Spinach and Bell Pepper

VEGETARIAN, GLUTEN FREE, DAIRY FREE
PREP TIME: 10 MIN **COOK TIME:** 20 MIN **SERVINGS:** 4
Calories: 130, Carbs: 22g, Fat: 4g, Protein: 5g, Fiber: 7g, Sodium: 15mg

- 2 large zucchinis, halved and hollowed
- 1 cup cooked lentils
- 1 cup diced tomatoes
- 1 tbsp olive oil
- 1 tsp dried oregano
- ½ cup fresh spinach, chopped
- ½ red bell pepper, diced

1. Turn the oven on to 375°F, or 190°C.
2. Combine the lentils, red bell pepper, spinach, diced tomatoes, oregano, and olive oil in a bowl.
3. Fill the zucchini hollows with the mixture.
4. After placing the filled zucchini on a baking dish, bake it for 20 minutes, or until the zucchini is soft and the filling is thoroughly heated.
5. Warm up and serve.

Mediterranean Roasted Asparagus Medley

VEGETARIAN, GLUTEN FREE, DAIRY FREE
PREP TIME: 05 MIN **COOK TIME:** 15 MIN **SERVINGS:** 4
Calories: 75, Carbs: 7g, Fat: 5g, Protein: 3g, Fiber: 3g, Sodium: 120mg

- 1 bunch asparagus, trimmed
- 1 tbsp olive oil
- 1 tbsp balsamic vinegar
- 1 pinch salt
- 1 pinch black pepper
- ½ cup cherry tomatoes, halved
- ½ cup zucchini, sliced
- 2 cloves garlic, minced
- 2 tbsp pine nuts

1. Set the oven's temperature to 400°F, or 200°C.
2. Add the asparagus, olive oil, balsamic vinegar, salt, and black pepper to a mixing bowl. Toss to coat the asparagus evenly.

3. Toss once more after adding the cherry tomatoes, sliced zucchini, and minced garlic to the bowl.
4. On a baking sheet, arrange the asparagus and vegetable mixture in a single layer. Roast until soft and beginning to caramelize, 12 to 15 minutes.
5. Sprinkle the pine nuts on top of the vegetables during the final two minutes of roasting, then put the oven back on to lightly toast them.
6. Take it out of the oven, serve it hot, and savor the mix of flavors!

Rosemary-Parsnip Bake with Almond Crust

VEGETARIAN, GLUTEN FREE, DAIRY FREE
PREP TIME: 10 MIN **COOK TIME:** 25 MIN **SERVINGS:** 4
Calories: 250, Carbs: 22g, Fat: 15g, Protein: 5g, Fiber: 6g, Sodium: 150mg

- 4 medium parsnips, peeled and cut into sticks
- 2 tbsp olive oil
- 1 tsp fresh rosemary, chopped
- ¼ cup almond flour
- ¼ cup plant-based Parmesan cheese
- 2 tbsp Dijon mustard
- ¼ cup unsweetened almond milk
- 1 pinch salt
- 1 pinch black pepper

1. Preheat the oven to 400°F (200°C). Line a baking sheet with parchment paper.
2. In a large bowl, toss the parsnip sticks with olive oil, rosemary, salt, and black pepper. Set aside.
3. In another bowl, whisk together the almond flour, plant-based Parmesan, Dijon mustard, and almond milk until it forms a thick, smooth paste.
4. Dip each parsnip stick into the almond-mustard mixture, ensuring it is evenly coated.
5. Arrange the coated parsnip sticks in a single layer on the prepared baking sheet.
6. Roast in the preheated oven for 20 to 25 minutes, turning the parsnips halfway through, until they are golden brown and crispy on the edges.
7. Remove from the oven and transfer the roasted parsnips to a serving platter. Serve warm and enjoy!

Savory Caramelized Onion & Mushroom Medley

VEGETARIAN, GLUTEN FREE, DAIRY FREE
PREP TIME: 05 MIN **COOK TIME:** 15 MIN **SERVINGS:** 4
Calories: 90, Carbs: 9g, Fat: 5g, Protein: 2g, Fiber: 2g, Sodium: 10mg

- 2 large onions, thinly sliced
- 250g button mushrooms, sliced
- 1 cup cherry tomatoes, halved
- 2 cups fresh spinach
- 2 tbsp olive oil
- 1 pinch salt
- 1 pinch thyme (optional)
- 1 tbsp balsamic glaze

1. Heat the olive oil in a large skillet over medium heat.
2. Add the onions and cook, turning often, until golden brown and caramelized, about 10 minutes.
3. Cook for a further five minutes, or until the mushrooms are soft, after adding the cherry tomatoes and mushrooms.
4. Add the spinach and cook for about two minutes, or until it has wilted.
5. If desired, garnish with salt and thyme and drizzle with balsamic glaze.
6. Take off the heat and use as a garnish or side dish for other foods.

Stir-Fried Snap Peas with Sesame and Mushrooms

VEGETARIAN, GLUTEN FREE, DAIRY FREE
PREP TIME: 10 MIN **COOK TIME:** 10 MIN **SERVINGS:** 4
Calories: 120, Carbs: 8g, Fat: 8g, Protein: 4g, Fiber: 3g, Sodium: 290mg

- 2 cups snap peas, trimmed
- 1 cup shiitake mushrooms, sliced
- 1 tbsp sesame oil
- ¼ cup red bell pepper, thinly sliced
- 1 tsp toasted sesame seeds
- 1 tbsp tamari or soy sauce

1. In a large skillet, heat the sesame oil over medium heat. Cook the mushrooms and red bell pepper for 5 minutes, or until the mushrooms are tender.
2. Add tamari and snap peas into pan for a further four to five minutes, or until they are crisp-tender.
3. Before serving, sprinkle with sesame seeds.

Cinnamon-Spiced Roasted Carrots with Sweet Potato, Parsnips and Chili

VEGETARIAN, GLUTEN FREE, DAIRY FREE
PREP TIME: 05 MIN **COOK TIME:** 20 MIN **SERVINGS:** 4
Calories: 60, Carbs: 10g, Fat: 3g, Protein: 1g, Fiber: 3g, Sodium: 5mg

- 4 medium carrots, peeled and sliced
- 2 medium sweet potatoes, peeled and diced
- 2 medium parsnips, peeled and sliced
- 1 small red chili, finely chopped
- 1 red onion, sliced
- 1 tbsp olive oil
- 1 tsp ground cinnamon
- 1 pinch salt
- 1 pinch paprika

1. Set the oven's temperature to 400°F, or 200°C.
2. Carrots, sweet potatoes, parsnips, red onion, olive oil, ground cinnamon, salt, paprika, and chopped chili should all be combined in a bowl. To ensure even coating, toss well.
3. On a baking sheet, arrange the vegetables in a single layer. Roast until soft and beginning to caramelize, stirring halfway through, 20 minutes.
4. Take out of the oven and serve hot.

Spaghetti Squash with Spinach and Pine Nuts

VEGETARIAN, GLUTEN FREE, DAIRY FREE
PREP TIME: 15 MIN **COOK TIME:** 20 MIN **SERVINGS:** 4
Calories: 210, Carbs: 20g, Fat: 14g, Protein: 4g, Fiber: 5g, Sodium: 60mg

- 1 medium spaghetti squash
- 2 cups fresh spinach, chopped
- ¼ cup pine nuts
- ½ cup cherry tomatoes, halved
- 2 cloves garlic, minced
- 2 tbsp olive oil
- ¼ tsp nutmeg
- Salt and pepper, to taste

1. Set the oven's temperature to 400°F, or 200°C. Remove the seeds from the spaghetti squash after slicing it in half.
2. Drizzle with olive oil, season with salt and pepper, and roast for 20 to 25 minutes, or until the meat is tender and the strands come apart easily with a fork.
3. Toast the pine nuts in a small pan over medium heat for three to four minutes, or until they are golden brown. Put aside.
4. On a baking sheet, roast the garlic and cherry tomatoes with a little olive oil for 10 minutes, or until they are tender.
5. When the squash is cooked, scoop the strands into a big bowl and add the garlic, roasted cherry tomatoes, toasted pine nuts, spinach, and nutmeg. If preferred, add a bit more olive oil and toss softly. Warm up and serve.

Roasted Kohlrabi with Almond Crumble

VEGETARIAN, GLUTEN FREE, DAIRY FREE
PREP TIME: 05 MIN **COOK TIME:** 25 MIN **SERVINGS:** 4
Calories: 190, Carbs: 20g, Fat: 12g, Protein: 5g, Fiber: 7g, Sodium: 120mg

- 2 medium kohlrabi bulbs
- ¼ cup almond meal
- 1 tbsp tahini
- 1 tsp lemon juice
- 2 tbsp olive oil
- 1 tsp smoked paprika
- 1 tbsp fresh thyme leaves (or 1 tsp dried thyme)
- Salt and pepper, to taste
- 1 tbsp fresh parsley, chopped (for garnish)

1. Set the oven's temperature to 400°F, or 200°C. Put parchment paper on a baking pan.
2. Cut the kohlrabi bulbs into cubes after peeling them. Add salt, pepper, smoked paprika, thyme, and olive oil. Arrange the cubes in a single layer on the baking sheet.
3. To give the kohlrabi cubes more texture and taste, sprinkle them with almond meal. Make sure the coating is uniform.
4. The kohlrabi should be soft and golden brown after 20 to 25 minutes of roasting, with a midway turn.
5. Make the Lemon Tahini Drizzle: In a small bowl, combine the tahini and lemon juice while the kohlrabi roasts. To get a smooth, drizzle-able consistency, add a little water.
6. After taking the roasted kohlrabi out of the oven, place it on a platter. Garnish with fresh parsley and drizzle with the lemon-tahini sauce.
7. Serve hot

Grilled Artichokes with Rosemary

VEGETARIAN, GLUTEN FREE, DAIRY FREE
PREP TIME: 10 MIN **COOK TIME:** 20 MIN **SERVINGS:** 2
Calories: 160, Carbs: 18g, Fat: 8g, Protein: 4g, Fiber: 7g, Sodium: 40mg

- 2 large artichokes, halved and trimmed
- 1 tbsp olive oil
- ½ cup steamed green beans, chopped
- ¼ cup sun-dried tomatoes, chopped
- 2 tbsp pine nuts
- 2 tsp balsamic vinegar
- 1 tbsp fresh oregano, chopped
- 1 tbsp fresh rosemary, chopped

1. Cut off the tops of the artichokes and remove the tough outer leaves to trim them. Cut them in half, then take out the fuzzy choke.
2. Steam or boil the artichokes for 15-20 minutes until soft, then drain them thoroughly.
3. In a small bowl, mix olive oil, balsamic vinegar, chopped green beans, sun-dried tomatoes, and pine nuts. Brush this mixture over the artichokes, ensuring they are evenly coated.
4. Preheat your grill to medium-high heat. Grill the artichokes cut side down for 5-7 minutes, or until crispy and browned on the edges.
5. Serve immediately, optionally topping with extra pine nuts or sun-dried tomatoes for added texture and flavor. Enjoy!

Braised Fennel with Pistachios

VEGETARIAN, GLUTEN FREE, DAIRY FREE
PREP TIME: 05 MIN **COOK TIME:** 25 MIN **SERVINGS:** 4
Calories: 220, Carbs: 14g, Fat: 16g, Protein: 4g, Fiber: 4g, Sodium: 100mg

- 2 medium fennel bulbs, sliced
- ½ cup canned coconut cream
- ¼ cup vegetable broth
- ¼ cup crushed pistachios
- ½ cup frozen green peas
- 1 tbsp olive oil
- 1 tsp ground coriander
- 1 pinch salt
- 1 pinch black pepper

1. In a skillet, heat the olive oil over medium heat. Cook the sliced fennel for five minutes, or until it starts to caramelize a little.
2. Add the coconut cream and veggie broth. Add salt, pepper, and ground coriander and stir. The fennel should be soft after 15 to 20 minutes of simmering under cover.
3. In the final five minutes of simmering, stir in the green peas.
4. Crushed pistachios should be sprinkled on top after transferring to a serving dish.
5. Serve warm as a rich and creamy side dish or main entrée.

Stuffed Acorn Squash with Quinoa & Tomatoes

VEGETARIAN, GLUTEN FREE, DAIRY FREE
PREP TIME: 05 MIN **COOK TIME:** 25 MIN **SERVINGS:** 4
Calories: 200, Carbs: 15g, Fat: 10g, Protein: 6g, Fiber: 4g, Sodium: 120mg

- 2 medium acorn squash, halved and seeds scooped out
- 1 cup cooked quinoa
- 1 cup cherry tomatoes, halved
- ½ cup cooked chickpeas
- ¼ cup sunflower seeds (or pine nuts)
- 1 tsp ground cumin
- ½ tsp smoked paprika
- 1 tbsp olive oil
- Salt and black pepper, to taste

1. Preheat the oven to 375°F (190°C). Place the acorn squash halves, cut side up, on a baking sheet. Drizzle with olive oil, and season with salt, black pepper, cumin, and smoked paprika. Roast for 20-25 minutes, until the squash is tender.
2. While the squash is roasting, combine the cooked quinoa, halved cherry tomatoes, chickpeas, and sunflower seeds in a bowl. Add salt and black pepper to taste.
3. Once the squash is done, scoop the quinoa mixture into the squash halves.
4. Return the stuffed squash to the oven for another 5-7 minutes to heat through.
5. Serve warm and enjoy the flavorful, wholesome meal!

Spaghetti Squash with Tomato and Basil Sauce

VEGETARIAN, GLUTEN FREE, DAIRY FREE
PREP TIME: 10 MIN **COOK TIME:** 20 MIN **SERVINGS:** 4
Calories: 130, Carbs: 20g, Fat: 6g, Protein: 4g, Fiber: 5g, Sodium: 160mg

- 1 medium spaghetti squash, cooked
- 2 cups cherry tomatoes, halved
- ¼ cup tomato paste
- 2 tbsp olive oil
- 1 medium zucchini, diced
- ½ tsp garlic powder
- Fresh basil leaves, for garnish

1. Heat olive oil in a pan over medium heat. Add cherry tomatoes and cook for 5 minutes until softened.
2. Add diced zucchini and cook for another 3-4 minutes, until tender.
3. Stir in tomato paste and ½ cup water. Simmer for 3-5 minutes until the sauce thickens. Season with salt, pepper, and garlic powder.
4. Add the cooked spaghetti squash to the sauce, mixing thoroughly to combine.
5. Serve with fresh basil leaves for garnish. Enjoy!

Roasted Bell Peppers with Olive Tapenade

VEGETARIAN, GLUTEN FREE, DAIRY FREE
PREP TIME: 05 MIN **COOK TIME:** 20 MIN **SERVINGS:** 4
Calories: 160, Carbs: 16g, Fat: 11g, Protein: 3g, Fiber: 7g, Sodium: 290mg

- 2 large bell peppers, halved and seeded
- 2 tbsp olive oil
- ¼ cup kalamata olives, chopped
- 1 tbsp capers, chopped
- ½ cup cherry tomatoes, halved
- 2 tbsp sunflower seeds, toasted
- 1 tbsp lemon juice
- 1 pinch black pepper

1. Preheat your oven to 400°F (200°C).
2. Place the bell pepper halves on a baking sheet, cut side up. Drizzle them with olive oil and sprinkle with a pinch of black pepper.
3. Roast the bell peppers in the oven for 15-20 minutes, or until the peppers are soft and slightly charred.
4. While the peppers are roasting, prepare the olive tapenade: in a bowl, combine the chopped kalamata olives, capers, cherry tomatoes, toasted sunflower seeds, and lemon juice. Mix everything together until well combined.
5. Once the bell peppers are roasted, remove them from the oven and let them cool slightly.
6. Spoon the olive tapenade mixture into each bell pepper half.
7. Serve immediately and enjoy!

Steamed Artichokes with Avocado Tahini Dressing

VEGETARIAN, GLUTEN FREE, DAIRY FREE
PREP TIME: 10 MIN **COOK TIME:** 25 MIN **SERVINGS:** 4
Calories: 220, Carbs: 15g, Fat: 17g, Protein: 3g, Fiber: 9g, Sodium: 180mg

- 4 medium artichokes, trimmed and halved
- 1 ripe avocado
- 2 tbsp tahini
- ¼ cup toasted pine nuts
- ½ cup chopped cucumber
- ¼ cup chopped fresh parsley
- 1 tbsp fresh lemon juice
- 1 tbsp olive oil
- Salt and pepper, to taste

1. Trim the top leaves and chop off the stems to prepare the artichokes. Slice them in half, then use a spoon to remove the choke.
2. In a large pot over simmering water, steam the artichokes for 25 to 30 minutes, or until they are soft. To test for softness, peel off a leaf; it should come off with ease.
3. While the artichokes are steaming, make the avocado tahini dressing: Put the ripe avocado, tahini, lemon juice, olive oil, salt, and pepper in a food processor or blender. Blend until creamy and smooth. Adjust the consistency by adding a small amount of water if necessary.
4. Once the artichokes are cooked, place them on a platter and cover with the avocado-tahini dressing.
5. Sprinkle the toasted pine nuts, chopped cucumber, and fresh parsley on top before serving.
6. Serve warm or at room temperature.

Miso Glazed Bok Choy

VEGETARIAN, GLUTEN FREE, DAIRY FREE
PREP TIME: 05 MIN **COOK TIME:** 10 MIN **SERVINGS:** 2
Calories: 120, Carbs: 10g, Fat: 8g, Protein: 3g, Fiber: 3g, Sodium: 250mg

- 4 baby bok choy, halved
- 2 tbsp miso paste
- 1 tbsp sesame oil
- ½ cup sliced shiitake mushrooms
- 1 tbsp rice vinegar
- 1 clove garlic, minced
- 1 tbsp grated ginger
- 1 tbsp coconut aminos

1. Put the miso paste, rice vinegar, sesame oil, grated ginger, coconut aminos, and garlic in a small bowl. Mix thoroughly.
2. A big skillet should be heated to medium heat.
3. Put the bok choy cut-side down and heat until it starts to sear, about 2 to 3 minutes.
4. Turn the bok choy over and add the shiitake mushrooms to the skillet. After adding the miso glaze, sauté the vegetables for a further three to four minutes, or until they are soft and the glaze has covered everything.
5. Pour any remaining glaze over the top after transferring to a serving plate. Warm up and serve.

Grilled Portobello Mushrooms on Spinach Bed with Balsamic Glaze

VEGETARIAN, GLUTEN FREE, DAIRY FREE
PREP TIME: 05 MIN **COOK TIME:** 10 MIN **SERVINGS:** 4
Calories: 70, Carbs: 6g, Fat: 4g, Protein: 2g, Fiber: 1g, Sodium: 40mg

- 4 large portobello mushrooms, cleaned and stems removed
- 2 tbsp balsamic vinegar
- ¼ cup chopped red onion
- ½ cup fresh spinach, chopped
- ¼ cup pine nuts
- 1 tbsp olive oil
- 1 pinch salt
- 1 pinch black pepper

1. Apply salt, pepper, balsamic vinegar, and olive oil to the mushrooms.
2. Turn the grill on to medium-high heat.
3. Grill the mushrooms for 5 minutes on each side until they are soft and gently browned.
4. After grilling, top the mushrooms with the chopped red onion, fresh spinach, and pine nuts.
5. Serve warm and enjoy!

Sautéed Celeriac with Shallots

VEGETARIAN, GLUTEN FREE, DAIRY FREE
PREP TIME: 05 MIN **COOK TIME:** 15 MIN **SERVINGS:** 4
Calories: 190, Carbs: 24g, Fat: 8g, Protein: 3g, Fiber: 8g, Sodium: 70mg

- 1 medium celeriac (celery root), peeled and diced
- 1 tbsp olive oil
- ¼ cup shallots, sliced
- ¼ cup chopped celery
- ¼ cup vegetable broth
- 1 tbsp fresh sage leaves, chopped
- 1 tbsp apple cider vinegar
- Salt and pepper, to taste

1. In a skillet, heat the olive oil over medium heat. Cook the shallots for 2 to 3 minutes, or until they are tender.
2. Add the chopped celery and cook for an additional 2 minutes, stirring frequently.
3. Add the diced celeriac to the skillet and cook for 8 to 10 minutes, or until it is soft and golden.
4. Pour in the vegetable broth, apple cider vinegar, and chopped sage. Stir well and cook for 2 more minutes until the mixture becomes aromatic.
5. Season with salt and pepper to taste. Serve warm

Swiss Chard Rolls Stuffed with Lentil Rice

VEGETARIAN, GLUTEN FREE, DAIRY FREE
PREP TIME: 10 MIN **COOK TIME:** 20 MIN **SERVINGS:** 4
Calories: 240, Carbs: 20g, Fat: 12g, Protein: 8g, Fiber: 6g, Sodium: 40mg

- 8 large Swiss chard leaves
- 1 cup cooked lentils
- ½ cup cooked brown rice
- ½ cup diced tomatoes
- ½ cup coconut cream
- 1 tbsp olive oil

1. For one minute, blanch the Swiss chard leaves in boiling water. Set aside after draining.
2. Put the cooked lentils, rice, diced tomatoes, and olive oil in a bowl.
3. Roll firmly after spooning the food into each Swiss chard leaf.
4. Put the rolls in a skillet, pour coconut cream over them, and let them boil for ten minutes.
5. Serve after warming up.

Sautéed Kale with Lemon and Garlic

VEGETARIAN, GLUTEN FREE, DAIRY FREE
PREP TIME: 05 MIN **COOK TIME:** 10 MIN **SERVINGS:** 4
Calories: 100, Carbs: 5g, Fat: 8g, Protein: 2g, Fiber: 2g, Sodium: 40mg

- 4 cups kale, stems removed and chopped
- 2 cloves garlic, minced
- 2 tbsp olive oil
- ¼ cup chopped walnuts
- ¼ cup roasted red peppers, chopped
- 1 tbsp hemp seeds
- 1 tbsp lemon juice
- 1 pinch salt

1. In a large skillet, heat the olive oil over medium heat.
2. Cook the garlic for one minute, or until it becomes aromatic.
3. Add the kale to the skillet and cook for 5 to 7 minutes, turning often, until it wilts.
4. Stir in the roasted red peppers and chopped walnuts for added flavor and crunch.
5. Before serving, drizzle with lemon juice and sprinkle with hemp seeds for a protein boost.

Grilled Eggplant and Roasted Pepper Stew

VEGETARIAN, GLUTEN FREE, DAIRY FREE
PREP TIME: 05 MIN **COOK TIME:** 20 MIN **SERVINGS:** 4
Calories: 145, Carbs: 15g, Fat: 9g, Protein: 4g, Fiber: 6g, Sodium: 85mg

- 2 medium eggplants, diced
- 2 tbsp olive oil
- 1 tsp dried thyme
- Salt and pepper, to taste
- ½ cup cherry tomatoes, halved
- ¼ cup roasted bell peppers, sliced
- ¼ cup pomegranate seeds
- 1 tbsp lemon juice
- ¼ cup feta cheese (dairy-free option: plant-based feta)

1. Heat the olive oil in a large pot over medium heat. Add the diced eggplant and cook for about 10 minutes, stirring occasionally, until the eggplant is tender and golden.
2. Add the cherry tomatoes and roasted bell peppers to the pot. Stir well and cook for an additional 5 minutes.
3. Season with salt, pepper, and dried thyme. Add a splash of water if needed to prevent sticking.
4. Remove from heat and stir in the lemon juice.
5. Top the stew with feta (or plant-based feta) and sprinkle with pomegranate seeds for a burst of sweetness.
6. Serve warm as a hearty, flavorful dish.

Creamy Cauliflower and Leek Mash

VEGETARIAN, GLUTEN FREE, DAIRY FREE
PREP TIME: 05 MIN **COOK TIME:** 20 MIN **SERVINGS:** 4
Calories: 140, Carbs: 18g, Fat: 7g, Protein: 3g, Fiber: 5g, Sodium: 80mg

- 1 medium cauliflower, cut into florets
- 2 medium leeks, cleaned and sliced
- 1 tbsp olive oil
- ¼ cup coconut milk (or any dairy-free milk)
- ½ tsp turmeric powder
- Salt and pepper, to taste
- Fresh chives, chopped, for garnish

1. Cook the cauliflower florets in a large pot with boiling water for 10 to 12 minutes, or until they are soft.
2. Heat the olive oil in a separate pan over medium heat. Sauté the leeks for five to seven minutes, or until they are tender and have a hint of caramel.
3. After draining, put the cauliflower in a food processor or blender. Stir in the coconut milk, turmeric, salt, pepper, and sautéed leeks.
4. Blend till creamy and smooth. To get the right consistency, add a little more coconut milk if the mixture is too thick.
5. Garnish with fresh chives and serve.

Spiced Cauliflower Rice with Peas, Carrots, and Cilantro

VEGETARIAN, GLUTEN FREE, DAIRY FREE
PREP TIME: 10 MIN **COOK TIME:** 15 MIN **SERVINGS:** 4
Calories: 130, Carbs: 15g, Fat: 7g, Protein: 3g, Fiber: 5g, Sodium: 150mg

- 2 cups cauliflower, grated into rice-like texture
- 1 tbsp olive oil
- ½ tsp ground turmeric
- ¼ tsp smoked paprika
- 1 pinch salt
- ½ cup frozen peas, thawed
- ½ cup grated carrots
- 2 tbsp fresh cilantro, chopped
- ½ tsp cumin seeds

1. Grate cauliflower or pulse in a food processor to create rice-like pieces.
2. Heat olive oil in a skillet over medium heat. Add cumin seeds and cook for 1 minute until fragrant.
3. Add the grated cauliflower, turmeric, smoked paprika, and salt to the skillet. Cook for 8-10 minutes, stirring occasionally, until the cauliflower is tender and begins to brown.
4. Stir in peas and grated carrots, and cook for another 3-5 minutes until the vegetables are softened.
5. Remove from heat, mix in fresh cilantro, adjust seasoning if needed, and serve warm

Zucchini Noodles with Almond Pesto and Roasted Vegetables

VEGETARIAN, GLUTEN FREE, DAIRY FREE
PREP TIME: 05 MIN **COOK TIME:** 05 MIN **SERVINGS:** 2
Calories: 180, Carbs: 15g, Fat: 14g, Protein: 4g, Fiber: 4g, Sodium: 55mg

- **2 medium zucchinis, spiralized**
- **2 tbsp almond pesto (homemade or store-bought)**
- **1 tbsp olive oil**
- **¼ tsp chili flakes (optional)**
- **1 tbsp lemon juice**
- **½ cup cherry tomatoes, halved**
- **¼ cup red bell pepper, sliced**
- **¼ cup roasted pumpkin, cubed**

1. Spiralize the zucchini into thin noodles and set aside.
2. Heat the olive oil in a big skillet over medium heat.
3. In the pan, add the roasted pumpkin, red bell pepper, and cherry tomatoes. Sauté for two to three minutes, or until the pumpkin is tender.
4. Sauté the zucchini noodles for two to three minutes, or until they are just starting to soften.
5. Remove the pan from the heat and combine the noodles, almond pesto, lemon juice, and chili flakes.
6. Garnish with additional chili flakes if desired, then plate and serve.

Stuffed Veggie Portobello Mushrooms

VEGETARIAN, GLUTEN FREE
PREP TIME: 05 MIN **COOK TIME:** 20 MIN **SERVINGS:** 2
Calories: 180, Carbs: 12g, Fat: 11g, Protein: 6g, Fiber: 4g, Sodium: 220mg

- **4 large Portobello mushrooms, stems removed**
- **½ cup cherry tomatoes, diced**
- **2 tbsp kalamata olives, chopped**
- **1 tbsp olive oil**
- **1 tbsp balsamic vinegar**
- **1 tsp dried oregano**
- **½ cup fresh spinach, chopped**
- **2 tbsp crumbled feta cheese**

1. Set the oven's temperature to 200°C (400°F).
2. Put the spinach, cherry tomatoes, olives, olive oil, oregano, and balsamic vinegar in a bowl.
3. Place the mushrooms on a baking pan and spoon the mixture into each mushroom cap.
4. The mushrooms should be cooked through and tender after 15 to 20 minutes in the oven.
5. As a main course, serve hot.

Braised Turnips with Miso and Scallions

VEGETARIAN, GLUTEN FREE, DAIRY FREE
PREP TIME: 05 MIN **COOK TIME:** 15 MIN **SERVINGS:** 4
Calories: 120, Carbs: 15g, Fat: 6g, Protein: 2g, Fiber: 3g, Sodium: 280mg

- **4 medium turnips, peeled and quartered**
- **1 tbsp white miso paste**
- **½ cup vegetable broth**
- **¼ cup scallions, sliced**
- **¼ cup diced carrots**
- **1 tbsp sesame oil**
- **Salt and pepper**

1. In a skillet, heat the sesame oil over medium heat. Cook the turnips for around five minutes, or until they are gently browned and set aside.
2. Mix the miso paste and vegetable broth together. Add the mixture to the turnips and carrots, then simmer covered for 10 minutes, or until the turnips are soft.
3. Take off the top, add the scallions, and continue cooking for another minute.
4. Warm up and serve as a light main course or side dish.

Cauliflower and Spinach Stir-Fry with Almond

VEGETARIAN, GLUTEN FREE, DAIRY FREE
PREP TIME: 05 MIN **COOK TIME:** 20 MIN **SERVINGS:** 2
Calories: 150, Carbs: 14g, Fat: 10g, Protein: 5g, Fiber: 6g, Sodium: 40mg

- 2 cups cauliflower florets
- 2 cups spinach, washed
- 1 tbsp olive oil
- 1 tsp turmeric
- ½ cup diced carrots
- 2 cloves garlic, minced
- ¼ cup sliced almonds
- ½ tsp ground cumin
- ½ tsp smoked paprika
- Salt and pepper, to taste

1. Heat olive oil in a large skillet over medium heat. Add cauliflower florets and sauté for 8 to 10 minutes until tender and golden.
2. Add minced garlic and diced carrots, cooking for an additional 2 to 3 minutes, or until fragrant and the carrots begin to soften.
3. Stir in spinach and turmeric, cooking for another 5 to 7 minutes until the spinach wilts and cauliflower is fully cooked.
4. Season with cumin, smoked paprika, salt, and pepper. Stir in the sliced almonds for a crunchy texture just before serving.
5. Remove from heat and serve immediately. Enjoy!

Roasted Brussels Sprouts with Lemon and Garlic

VEGETARIAN, GLUTEN FREE, DAIRY FREE
PREP TIME: 05 MIN **COOK TIME:** 25 MIN **SERVINGS:** 4
Calories: 180, Carbs: 22g, Fat: 12g, Protein: 6g, Fiber: 7g, Sodium: 100mg

- 2 cups Brussels sprouts, trimmed and halved
- 2 tbsp olive oil
- 2 cloves garlic, minced
- 1 tbsp lemon juice
- ¼ cup dried cranberries
- ¼ cup chopped pecans
- ½ cup roasted chickpeas
- 1 pinch salt
- 1 pinch black pepper

1. Set the oven's temperature to 400°F (200°C).
2. Add salt, pepper, lemon juice, garlic, and olive oil to the Brussels sprouts and toss to coat.
3. Spread the Brussels sprouts on a baking sheet and roast for 25 minutes, or until golden brown and crispy.
4. During the last 5 minutes of roasting, sprinkle the dried cranberries, chopped pecans, and roasted chickpeas over the Brussels sprouts.
5. Once done, remove from the oven and serve warm.

Steamed Broccolini with Sesame Dressing

VEGETARIAN, GLUTEN FREE, DAIRY FREE
PREP TIME: 05 MIN **COOK TIME:** 10 MIN **SERVINGS:** 4
Calories: 70, Carbs: 4g, Fat: 5g, Protein: 2g, Fiber: 2g, Sodium: 60mg

- 1 bunch broccolini, trimmed
- 1 tbsp sesame oil
- 1 tsp soy sauce (or tamari for gluten-free)
- ½ cup shredded carrots
- ¼ cup chopped scallions
- 1 tbsp rice vinegar
- 1 tsp sesame seeds

1. After 5 to 7 minutes of steaming, the broccolini should be tender but still bright green.
2. Put the rice vinegar, sesame oil, and soy sauce in a small bowl.
3. Top the steamed broccolini with chopped scallions, sesame seeds, and shredded carrots.
4. Serve right away after adding a drizzle of the sesame dressing.

Stuffed Tomatoes with Lentils and Herbs

VEGETARIAN, GLUTEN FREE, DAIRY FREE
PREP TIME: 05 MIN **COOK TIME:** 20 MIN **SERVINGS:** 2
Calories: 210, Carbs: 20g, Fat: 8g, Protein: 9g, Fiber: 6g, Sodium: 120mg

- 4 large tomatoes, tops removed and insides scooped out
- 1 cup cooked green lentils
- ¼ cup vegan feta cheese
- ¼ cup chopped parsley
- ½ cup cooked rice
- 2 tbsp olive oil
- 1 tsp smoked paprika
- 1 pinch salt
- 1 pinch black pepper

1. Turn the oven on to 375°F, or 190°C. Olive oil should be lightly brushed over the hollowed-out tomatoes.
2. Combine the cooked rice, lentils, vegan feta, smoked paprika, parsley, salt, and pepper in a bowl.
3. Fill the hollowed-out tomatoes with the filling using a spoon. On a baking sheet, arrange them.

4. The tomatoes should be soft and faintly caramelized after 15 to 20 minutes in the oven.
5. As a tasty main meal, serve hot.

Roasted Vegetables with Honey Lemon Glaze

VEGETARIAN, GLUTEN FREE, DAIRY FREE
PREP TIME: 10 MIN **COOK TIME:** 25 MIN **SERVINGS:** 4
Calories: 190, Carbs: 22g, Fat: 7g, Protein: 3g, Fiber: 6g, Sodium: 35mg

- **2 large fennel bulbs, trimmed and sliced into wedges**
- **2 medium carrots, peeled and sliced into sticks**
- **1 small butternut squash, peeled, seeded, and cubed**
- **1 medium zucchini, sliced into rounds**
- **2 tbsp olive oil**
- **1 tbsp honey (or maple syrup for vegan option)**
- **1 tbsp lemon juice**
- **1 tsp lemon zest**

1. Preheat your oven to 400°F (200°C). Line a baking sheet with parchment paper.
2. In a large bowl, toss the fennel, butternut squash, zucchini, and carrots with olive oil until evenly coated. Spread them out on the baking sheet in a single layer.
3. Roast in the oven for 20–25 minutes, flipping halfway through, until the vegetables are caramelized and tender.
4. In a small bowl, whisk together the honey (or maple syrup), lemon juice, and lemon zest.
5. Remove the vegetables from the oven and drizzle the honey-lemon glaze over them. Toss gently to coat.
6. Serve warm, garnished with additional lemon zest, if desired.

Coconut Turmeric Vegetable Stew

VEGETARIAN, GLUTEN FREE, DAIRY FREE
PREP TIME: 05 MIN **COOK TIME:** 25 MIN **SERVINGS:** 2
Calories: 220, Carbs: 20g, Fat: 13g, Protein: 4g, Fiber: 6g, Sodium: 150mg

- **2 medium turnips, peeled and cubed**
- **2 medium carrots, sliced**
- **1 cup coconut milk**
- **1 cup green beans, trimmed and halved**
- **1 cup vegetable broth**
- **2 tbsp olive oil**
- **1 tsp ground turmeric**
- **1 tsp ground cumin**
- **½ tsp smoked paprika**
- **Salt and pepper, to taste**

1. Heat olive oil in a large pot over medium heat. Add the turnips and carrots, cooking for 5 minutes while stirring occasionally.
2. Add turmeric, cumin, and smoked paprika to the pot. Stir well to coat the vegetables with the spices and cook for 1-2 minutes until fragrant.
3. Pour in the vegetable broth and coconut milk. Bring to a boil, then reduce heat to a simmer and cook for 10 minutes.
4. Add the green beans and simmer for an additional 10 minutes, or until all vegetables are tender.
5. Season with salt and black pepper to taste. Serve warm with a sprinkle of smoked paprika for garnish if desired.

Caramelized Rutabaga with Miso Glaze

VEGETARIAN, GLUTEN FREE, DAIRY FREE
PREP TIME: 05 MIN **COOK TIME:** 20 MIN **SERVINGS:** 4
Calories: 190, Carbs: 14g, Fat: 12g, Protein: 2g, Fiber: 5g, Sodium: 120mg

- **2 medium rutabagas, peeled and cubed**
- **2 tbsp white miso paste**
- **1 tbsp maple syrup**
- **2 tbsp sesame oil**
- **2 green onions, sliced**
- **1 tsp sesame seeds (optional, for garnish)**

1. In a large skillet, heat the sesame oil over medium heat. Cook the rutabaga cubes for 10 minutes, stirring periodically, until they are lightly browned.
2. In a small bowl, combine the white miso paste, maple syrup, and 2 tablespoons of water. Add the miso mixture to the skillet and toss the rutabaga to ensure it is evenly coated.
3. Continue cooking for another 10 minutes, or until the rutabaga is soft and the glaze has thickened.
4. Sprinkle the sliced green onions on top just before serving for added crunch and flavor.
5. If preferred, top with sesame seeds before serving.

Braised Leeks with Almonds and Chickpeas

VEGETARIAN, GLUTEN FREE, DAIRY FREE
PREP TIME: 05 MIN **COOK TIME:** 25 MIN **SERVINGS:** 4
Calories: 220, Carbs: 18g, Fat: 10g, Protein: 7g, Fiber: 4g, Sodium: 90mg

- 3 medium leeks, sliced lengthwise
- 1 cup canned chickpeas, drained and rinsed
- ¼ cup slivered almonds
- ¼ cup vegetable broth
- ½ cup unsweetened almond milk
- 2 tbsp olive oil
- 1 tsp ground cumin
- 1 pinch salt
- 1 pinch black pepper

1. In a skillet, heat the olive oil over medium heat. Cook the leeks for five minutes, or until they are just beginning to soften.
2. Add almond milk and veggie broth. Add the ground cumin, chickpeas, salt, and pepper and stir. Simmer for 15 minutes with a lid on.
3. Remove the cover and top with sliced almonds. Cook until the leeks are soft and the almonds are just beginning to roast, about 5 more minutes.
4. Drizzle the braising liquid over the warm dish.

Braised Fennel with White Beans and Tomatoes

VEGETARIAN, GLUTEN FREE, DAIRY FREE
PREP TIME: 10 MIN **COOK TIME:** 25 MIN **SERVINGS:** 2
Calories: 160, Carbs: 21g, Fat: 5g, Protein: 6g, Fiber: 7g, Sodium: 120mg

- 2 medium fennel bulbs, trimmed and sliced
- 1 cup canned white beans, drained and rinsed
- 1 cup cherry tomatoes, halved
- 1 tbsp tomato paste
- ½ cup vegetable broth
- 1 tsp smoked paprika
- 1 tbsp olive oil
- Salt and pepper, to taste

1. In a large skillet, heat the olive oil over medium heat. Cook the sliced fennel for five minutes, or until it starts to caramelize a little.
2. To the skillet, add the tomato paste, smoked paprika, white beans, and cherry tomatoes. Mix to blend.
3. Add the vegetable broth. Lower the heat to low, cover, and simmer until the fennel is soft and the sauce has thickened, 15 to 20 minutes.
4. Taste and adjust the salt and pepper. Serve warm as a filling side dish or main course.

Leeks with Mustard Cream Sauce

VEGETARIAN, GLUTEN FREE, DAIRY FREE
PREP TIME: 05 MIN **COOK TIME:** 20 MIN **SERVINGS:** 4
Calories: 80, Carbs: 10g, Fat: 5g, Protein: 2g, Fiber: 2g, Sodium: 85mg

- 3 large leeks, cleaned and sliced
- 2 tbsp olive oil
- 1 tbsp Dijon mustard
- 1 cup unsweetened almond milk
- 1 cup vegetable broth
- 1 tsp smoked paprika
- Salt and pepper, to taste

1. In a large skillet, heat the olive oil over medium heat. Cook the leeks for five minutes, or until they are just beginning to turn golden.
2. Add the vegetable broth, cover, and boil the leeks until they are soft, about 10 minutes.
3. Whisk the Dijon mustard and almond milk together in a small bowl. Combine this mixture with the leeks in a skillet.
4. Season with salt, pepper, and smoked paprika. Allow the sauce to slightly thicken by cooking it uncovered for an additional five minutes.
5. Spoon the creamy sauce over the leeks and serve warm as a light main course or as a side dish.

Fennel and Radish Slaw

VEGETARIAN, GLUTEN FREE, DAIRY FREE
PREP TIME: 10 MIN **COOK TIME:** 00 MIN **SERVINGS:** 4
Calories: 70, Carbs: 6g, Fat: 3g, Protein: 1g, Fiber: 2g, Sodium: 20mg

- 2 cups fennel, thinly sliced
- 1 cup radishes, thinly sliced
- 2 tbsp olive oil
- ¼ cup chopped fresh parsley
- ¼ cup sliced almonds
- 1 tbsp lemon juice
- ¼ cup shredded carrots
- 1 tbsp apple cider vinegar
- 1 pinch salt

1. In a mixing bowl, combine the radishes, fennel, and shredded carrots.

2. In a small bowl, whisk together the salt, apple cider vinegar, olive oil, and lemon juice.
3. Toss the vegetables thoroughly after adding the dressing.
4. Sprinkle with chopped parsley and sliced almonds for extra flavor and crunch.
5. Serve right away or refrigerate before serving.

Grilled Delicata Squash with Hazelnuts and Orange Zest

VEGETARIAN, GLUTEN FREE, DAIRY FREE
PREP TIME: 10 MIN **COOK TIME:** 15 MIN **SERVINGS:** 4
Calories: 180, Carbs: 27g, Fat: 9g, Protein: 3g, Fiber: 7g, Sodium: 55mg

- 2 delicata squash, sliced into rings
- 1 tbsp olive oil
- ¼ cup hazelnuts, chopped
- 1 tbsp orange zest
- 1 tbsp balsamic vinegar
- 1 tbsp maple syrup
- Salt and pepper, to taste

1. Set the grill's temperature to medium-high. Season the delicata squash rings with salt and pepper after drizzling them with olive oil.
2. The squash rings should be soft and browned after 8 to 10 minutes on each side of the grill.
3. Toast the chopped hazelnuts in a dry skillet over medium heat for two to three minutes, or until golden brown, while the squash is grilling.
4. Drizzle the balsamic vinegar and maple syrup over the grilled squash. Garnish with toasted hazelnuts and orange zest.
5. If preferred, top with additional salt and pepper and serve right away.

Celery Root Steaks with Capers and Dill

VEGETARIAN, GLUTEN FREE, DAIRY FREE
PREP TIME: 05 MIN **COOK TIME:** 20 MIN **SERVINGS:** 4
Calories: 160, Carbs: 18g, Fat: 9g, Protein: 3g, Fiber: 5g, Sodium: 310mg

- 1 large celery root (celeriac), peeled and sliced into 1-inch thick rounds
- 2 tbsp capers
- 1 tbsp fresh dill, chopped
- 2 tbsp olive oil
- ¼ cup vegetable broth
- ¼ cup sun-dried tomatoes, chopped
- ¼ cup olives, pitted and sliced
- Salt and pepper, to taste

1. In a large skillet, heat the olive oil over medium heat. Slices of celery root should be seared for three minutes on each side, or until golden brown.
2. Add vegetable broth, cover, and simmer until the celery root is soft, 12 to 15 minutes.
3. Add sun-dried tomatoes and olives to the pan, mixing gently.
4. Add fresh dill and capers on top as garnish. Add salt and pepper for seasoning.
5. As a main course or a side dish, serve hot.

Artichoke Hearts with Spinach-Almond Filling

VEGETARIAN, GLUTEN FREE, DAIRY FREE
PREP TIME: 15 MIN **COOK TIME:** 15 MIN **SERVINGS:** 4
Calories: 170, Carbs: 12g, Fat: 11g, Protein: 5g, Fiber: 6g, Sodium: 115mg

- 8 canned artichoke hearts, drained
- 1 cup fresh spinach, chopped
- ¼ cup almond flour
- 2 tbsp olive oil
- ¼ cup chopped olives (Kalamata or green)
- 2 tbsp nutritional yeast

1. Preheat the oven to 375°F (190°C) and lightly grease a baking dish.
2. Heat the olive oil in a skillet and cook the spinach until it wilts. Add nutritional yeast and almond flour to create a paste.
3. Stir in the chopped olives into the spinach-almond mixture.
4. Stuff each artichoke heart with the spinach-almond-olive mixture and place them on the prepared baking dish.
5. Bake for 15 to 20 minutes, or until lightly browned on top.
6. If preferred, top with more nutritional yeast and serve warm.

CHAPTER 8

WHOLEGRAINS, BEANS AND PASTA

Explore the Mediterranean's rich world of wholegrains, beans, and pasta! From filling grain salads to hearty stews and comforting pasta dishes, this chapter is packed with recipes that celebrate the heart of Mediterranean cooking—simple, fresh, and full of flavor. Let's dig in!

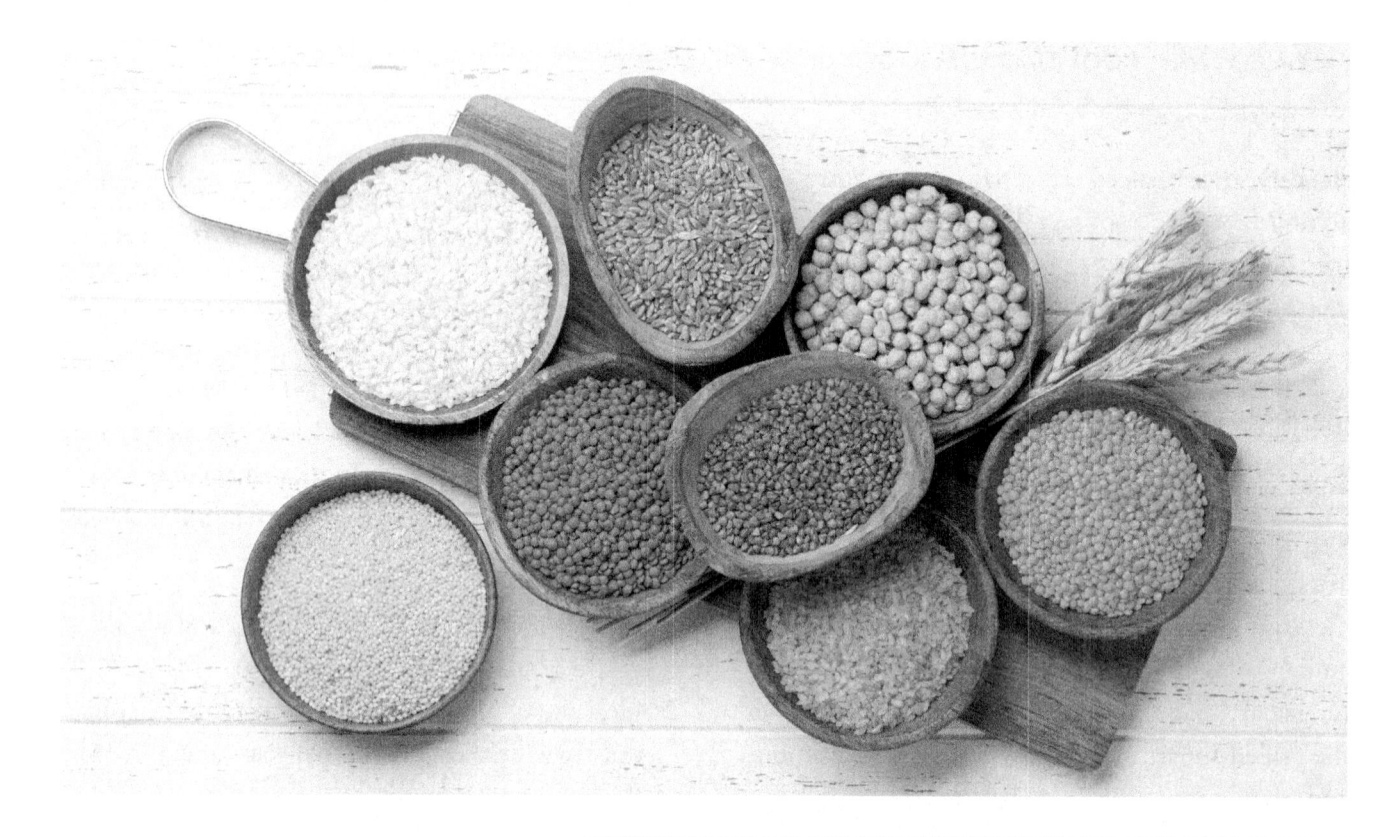

TIPS

- Swap grains like quinoa, farro, or barley to find your perfect flavor.

- Canned beans are a quick, protein-packed addition to any dish.

- Save some pasta water—it's the secret to a silky, flavorful sauce!

Crispy Persian Rice

VEGETARIAN

PREP TIME: 05 MIN **COOK TIME:** 25 MIN **SERVINGS:** 6

Calories: 314, Carbs: 49g, Protein: 5g, Fat: 5g, Fiber: 3g, Sodium: 321mg

- 1 cup warm water
- 1 tsp saffron threads
- 2 cups basmati rice
- 8 cups salted water
- 2 tbsp salt
- ¼ cup yogurt
- 2 tbsp seed oil
- 1 cup dried cherries
- 1 orange zest
- ½ tsp ground cinnamon
- 4-8 tbsp unsalted butter
- 3 tbsp pistachios

1. In warm water, soak saffron for 10 minutes. Wash rice until the water runs mostly clear.
2. Boil salted water. Cook rice for 5-6 minutes, drain. Combine 1 cup cooked rice, yogurt, and saffron water.
3. In a nonstick pot, spread yogurt-rice mix, then plain rice.
4. Add cherries, zest, and cinnamon. Repeat layers.
5. Pour remaining saffron water over rice and top with butter. Cover pot with towel-wrapped lid.
6. Cook on low heat until golden at the bottom.
7. Invert onto a plate, garnish with cherries and pistachios.

Egyptian Fava Beans

VEGETARIAN, DAIRY FREE, GLUTEN FREE

PREP TIME: 15 MIN **COOK TIME:** 10 MIN **SERVINGS:** 4

Calories: 143, Carbs: 27g, Protein: 10g, Fat: 1g, Fiber: 8g, Sodium: 342mg

- 2 cans fava beans
- ½ cup water
- Salt to taste
- ½ tsp ground cumin
- 2 hot peppers, chopped
- 2 garlic cloves, chopped
- 1 juiced lemon
- Olive oil to taste
- 1 cup parsley
- 1 tomato, chopped

1. Heat fava beans, water, salt, and cumin in a skillet.
2. Mash with a fork or masher. Mash hot peppers and garlic. Stir in lemon juice.
3. Pour sauce over mashed beans. Drizzle with olive oil.
4. Top with parsley, tomato, and optional hot pepper slices.
5. Serve with pita, veggies, and olives.

Mediterranean Bowl with Quinoa, Hummus, and Harissa

VEGETARIAN

PREP TIME: 10 MIN **COOK TIME:** 15 MIN **SERVINGS:** 4

Calories: 325, Carbs: 31g, Protein: 12g, Fat: 19g, Fiber: 7g, Sodium: 445mg

- 1 cup tri-color quinoa
- 1 ¾ cups water
- Salt, to taste
- 1 ½ cups hummus
- 4-6 oz feta cheese
- ½ cup kalamata olives
- 1 cup artichoke hearts
- Olive oil, to taste
- Aleppo pepper, to taste

1. Combine quinoa, water, and salt in a saucepan. Bring to a boil, cover, and simmer.
2. Let sit for 10 minutes, then fluff. In bowls, add hummus in the center.
3. Divide quinoa, salad, feta, olives, harissa (optional), and artichokes. Drizzle with olive oil and season with Aleppo pepper or sumac.
4. Serve immediately.

Cranberry Apple Freekeh Stuffing

VEGETARIAN, DAIRY FREE

PREP TIME: 05 MIN **COOK TIME:** 20 MIN **SERVINGS:** 8

Calories: 230, Carbs: 28g, Protein: 3g, Fat: 4g, Fiber: 2g, Sodium: 432mg

- 8 oz freekeh
- water
- 1 onion
- Olive oil, to taste
- 2 celery sticks, chopped
- 2 apples, chopped
- 2 garlic cloves, chopped
- Salt, to taste
- Black pepper, to taste
- 1 tsp sweet paprika
- 1 tsp ground allspice
- ½ tsp ground cinnamon
- 2 cups vegetable broth
- 2 cups dried cranberries
- 3 scallions, trimmed and chopped
- 1 cup parsley leaves
- 1 cup walnut halves

1. Soak freekeh in water, rinse, and drain. Heat 2 tbsp olive oil in a skillet.
2. Sauté onions, celery, apples, and garlic. Stir in freekeh, salt, pepper, and spices.
3. Add broth, bring to a boil, then simmer on low.
4. Stir in cranberries, cover, and cook for 7-10 more minutes. Stir in scallions and parsley.
5. Garnish with walnuts. Serve.

Greek Lemon Rice

DAIRY FREE, VEGETARIAN

PREP TIME: 10 MIN **COOK TIME:** 20 MIN **SERVINGS:** 5

Calories: 145 Carbs: 18g, Protein: 3g, Fat: 6g, Fiber: 6g, Sodium: 189mg

- 2 cups long grain rice
- 3 tbsp extra virgin olive oil
- 1 onion, chopped
- 1 garlic clove, minced
- ½ cup orzo pasta
- 2 lemons, juiced
- 2 cups low sodium vegetable broth
- Salt, a pinch
- Handful parsley, chopped
- 1 tsp dill weed

1. Rinse and soak rice in cold water, then drain.
2. Heat olive oil in a pan, cook onions. Add garlic and orzo, cook until orzo is browned. Stir in rice.
3. Add lemon juice and broth, bring to a boil. Reduce heat, cover, and cook until rice is tender, and liquid is absorbed.
4. Let it sit covered.
5. Stir in parsley, dill, and lemon zest. Garnish with lemon slices. Enjoy!

Black Bean Avocado Quinoa Bowl

VEGETARIAN, GLUTEN FREE

PREP TIME: 10 MIN **COOK TIME:** 00 MIN **SERVINGS:** 1

Calories: 500, Carbs: 74g, Protein: 20g, Fat: 16g, Fiber: 20g, Sodium: 210mg

- ¾ cup black beans
- ⅔ cup cooked quinoa
- 1 tbsp lime juice
- ¼ cup hummus
- 2 tbsp chopped cilantro
- 3 tbsp Pico De Gallo
- ¼ diced avocado

1. Add beans and quinoa to a bowl. Mix lime juice, hummus, and water.
2. Drizzle hummus dressing over the beans and quinoa, then top with cilantro, Pico de Gallo, and avocado.

Scan this QR code to download recipes with vibrant, full-color photos -'**A Reference Book of 70 Classic Mediterranean Recipes with Full Colored Pictures**'

Beans and Greens over Polenta

VEGETARIAN

PREP TIME: 10 MIN **COOK TIME:** 20 MIN **SERVINGS:** 4

Calories: 350, Carbs: 55g, Protein: 10g, Fat: 10g, Fiber: 6g, Sodium: 170mg

- ½ cup onion, chopped
- ½ cup parsley
- 1 bunch Swiss chard, chopped
- 1 tbsp tomato paste
- 4 cups vegetable broth
- ½ cup milk
- 2 tbsp olive oil
- ½ cup olive oil
- ½ cup dill
- 2 can eyes peas
- 1 lemon, juiced
- 1 cup cornmeal
- 1 garlic clove, minced
- Salt and pepper, to taste

1. Sauté onion in olive oil. Add parsley, dill, and sauté.
2. Stir in Swiss chard, cook. Add beans, tomato paste, lemon juice, and seasoning.
3. Let it simmer. Boil water in a pot. Stir in cornmeal, reduce heat, and cook. Add milk, garlic, olive oil, salt, and pepper.
4. Stir. Serve polenta with beans and greens on top.

Green Beans and Potatoes

VEGETARIAN, GLUTEN FREE

PREP TIME: 10 MIN **COOK TIME:** 20 MIN **SERVINGS:** 4

Calories: 408, Carbs: 38g, Protein: 7g, Fat: 28g, Fiber: 8g, Sodium: 230mg

- 1 can diced tomatoes
- ½ cup, olive oil
- 1 zucchini
- 1 dill (bunch)
- ½ bunch parsley
- 1 tsp oregano
- 1 lb green beans
- 2 potatoes
- 1 ½ sliced onion
- Salt and pepper, to taste

1. Heat a large pot over medium heat. Add olive oil, diced tomatoes, and water. Stir well.
2. Add the remaining ingredients and stir thoroughly. Bring the mixture to a simmer, stirring occasionally to ensure everything is well combined.
3. Cover the pot with a lid and lower the heat to low. Let it simmer for 15 minutes. After 15 minutes, remove the lid and check the consistency.
4. Stir again before serving. Be cautious, as the food will be hot. Enjoy!

Lebanese Green Beans with Olive Oil

VEGETARIAN, GLUTEN FREE, DAIRY FREE
PREP TIME: 10 MIN **COOK TIME:** 20 MIN **SERVINGS:** 4
Calories: 210, Carbs: 26g, Protein: 6g, Fat: 11g, Fiber: 9g, Sodium: 187mg

- 3 tbsp olive oil
- 1 onion, chopped
- 4 garlic cloves, chopped
- ½ tsp pepper
- 1 tomato
- 2 ¼ lb green beans
- 3 tbsp tomato paste
- 1 tsp salt

1. Heat olive oil in a large skillet over medium heat.
2. Add onions and cook for 3-5 minutes. Add garlic, pepper, salt, tomatoes, and beans.
3. Stir to combine. Mix in the tomato paste mixture. Stir well. Cover and cook on low heat, stirring occasionally, until beans are tender.

Rigatoni with Creamy Ricotta and Spinach

VEGETARIAN
PREP TIME: 10 MIN **COOK TIME:** 10 MIN **SERVINGS:** 4
Calories: 471, Carbs: 45g, Protein: 15g, Fat: 10g, Fiber: 2g, Sodium: 315mg

- ½ lb Ricotta
- 3 tbsp olive oil
- 1 tsp vinegar
- 1 tsp salt
- 1 tsp grounded pepper
- 2 ½ oz spinach
- 8 oz rigatoni pasta
- 2 tbsp parmesan cheese

1. Blend ricotta, 2 tbsp olive oil, vinegar, salt, and pepper. Add warm water if needed.
2. Stir spinach into ricotta mixture.
3. Cook pasta, reserve some water, then drain.
4. Mix pasta with ricotta-spinach sauce, adding Parmesan and pasta water to smooth.
5. Serve topped with ricotta and black pepper.

Lentils and Rice with Caramelized Onions

VEGETARIAN, GLUTEN FREE, DAIRY FREE
PREP TIME: 05 MIN **COOK TIME:** 25 MIN **SERVINGS:** 5
Calories: 448, Carbs: 75g, Protein: 19g, Fat: 8g, Fiber: 20g, Sodium: 154mg

- 1 ½ cup lentils
- 2 ½ tbsp olive oil
- 3 ½ onions
- 1 cup basmati rice
- 1 tsp salt
- ½ tsp ground cumin
- ¼ tsp turmeric
- 2 cups vegetable broth

1. Drain soaked lentils and remove debris.
2. Boil lentils in water. Drain and set aside. In a pan, heat olive oil and fry onions over high heat for 10 minutes.
3. Reserve one-third of the onions. Add rice, salt, cumin, and turmeric to the remaining onions.
4. Fry until fragrant. Add lentils and vegetable broth. Boil until rice is tender.
5. Stir and top with reserved crispy onions before serving.

Risotto Radicchio and Gorgonzola

VEGETARIAN, DAIRY FREE
PREP TIME: 10 MIN **COOK TIME:** 20 MIN **SERVINGS:** 2
Calories: 640, Carbs: 68g, Protein: 17g, Fat: 29g, Fiber: 3g, Sodium: 340mg

- 4 cups vegetable stock
- 1 small head radicchio
- 2 tbsp olive oil
- ½ onion, chopped
- ⅔ cup risotto rice
- ½ cup white wine
- 3 oz Gorgonzola Dolce cheese
- ⅛ cup parmesan cheese, grated
- Salt and pepper, to taste

1. Bring stock to a simmer in a pot.
2. Slice radicchio into thin strips, dice the white part, and discard the root.
3. Heat olive oil in a skillet, sauté onions for a few minutes.
4. Add rice, toast for 30 seconds, then deglaze with white wine.
5. Add stock, once ladle at a time, stirring until absorbed before adding more.
6. After 10 minutes, stir in most of the radicchio (reserve some for garnish).
7. Continue adding stock and cooking until rice is tender.
8. Turn off heat, stir in Gorgonzola, Parmesan, salt, and pepper until creamy.
9. Serve immediately, garnishing with reserved radicchio.

Pasta with Chickpeas

VEGETARIAN
PREP TIME: 10 MIN **COOK TIME:** 25 MIN **SERVINGS:** 4
Calories: 538, Carbs: 74g, Protein: 38g, Fat: 16g,
Fiber: 6g, Sodium: 345mg

- ¼ cup olive oil
- 2 garlic cloves, crushed
- 1 celery stalk, diced
- 1 onion, diced
- 1 tbsp rosemary, minced
- 1 tsp red pepper flakes
- 1 can (15 oz) chickpeas
- 1 can (14 oz) chopped tomatoes
- 6 cups vegetable broth
- 1 parmesan rind, grated (for serving)
- Kosher salt
- 2 cups ditalini pasta

1. Heat olive oil, sauté garlic, celery, and onion. Add rosemary and chili and cook.
2. Add chickpeas, broth, and tomatoes. Simmer for 5 minutes.
3. Add broth and parmesan rind and simmer.
4. Add pasta and cook. Adjust seasoning.
5. Serve with olive oil and grated parmesan.

Tunisian Chickpea Stew

VEGETARIAN
PREP TIME: 10 MIN **COOK TIME:** 20 MIN **SERVINGS:** 4
Calories: 196, Carbs: 40g, Protein: 07g, Fat: 02g,
Fiber: 4g, Sodium: 586mg

- 2 cans (15 oz each) chickpeas
- ½ loaf rustic bread
- Olive oil
- 1 onion, chopped
- 3 garlic cloves, minced
- Kosher salt
- 1 tsp ground cumin
- ½ tsp coriander
- ½ tsp paprika
- 1 tsp harissa paste
- 2 lemons
- ½ cup parsley, chopped
- 2 green onions, chopped

1. In a saucepan, cover the chickpeas with water. Bring to a boil, then simmer until soft.
2. Broil torn bread with olive oil until golden. Cook onions, garlic, and spices in olive oil until tender.
3. Add sautéed onions to chickpeas with harissa, lemon juice, parsley, and olive oil.
4. Layer toasted bread in bowls, top with chickpea stew, drizzle with olive oil, harissa, and garnish with parsley and green onions.

Greek Baked Beans

VEGETARIAN, DAIRY FREE, GLUTEN FREE
PREP TIME: 10 MIN **COOK TIME:** 20 MIN **SERVINGS:** 4
Calories: 182, Carbs: 24g, Protein: 06g, Fat: 07g,
Fiber: 7g, Sodium: 249mg

- ½ onion, chopped
- 1 celery stalk, chopped
- 2 garlic cloves, minced
- Kosher salt
- 2 can tomatoes, diced
- 6 tbsp water
- ¼ cup parsley, chopped
- ½ tbsp thyme leaves
- ¼ tsp dried oregano
- ½ tsp red pepper flakes
- ¼ tsp ground black pepper
- ⅛ tsp ground cinnamon
- 1 dried bay leaf
- 1 can (15 oz) of butter beans
- Creamy feta cheese, crumbled
- Rustic bread

1. Preheat oven to 375°F. Sauté onion, celery, and garlic in 1/8 cup olive oil with ¼ tsp salt.
2. Add tomatoes, water, ¼ tsp salt, herbs, and spices. Stir in beans and cook for 5 mins.
3. Bake until golden. Finish with olive oil, parsley, and feta. Serve with bread.

Freekeh

VEGETARIAN, DAIRY FREE
PREP TIME: 03 MIN **COOK TIME:** 20 MIN **SERVINGS:** 6
Calories: 86, Carbs: 18g, Protein: 5g, Fat: 1g, Fiber: 2g, Sodium: 134mg

- 1 cup freekeh grains
- 2 ½ cups broth
- Salt, to taste
- Parsley for garnish

1. Pick over any debris and rinse the freekeh well. Combine freekeh and water/broth in a saucepan.
2. Bring to a boil, season with salt, then reduce heat and cover. Simmer until tender and chewy.
3. Drain any excess water and fluff with a fork.
4. Garnish with chopped parsley and serve.

Garbanzo Bean Pilaf

VEGETARIAN
PREP TIME: 05 MIN **COOK TIME:** 30 MIN **SERVINGS:** 6
Calories: 276, Carbs: 37g, Protein: 9g, Fat: 11g, Fiber: 7g, Sodium: 230mg

- 1 can garbanzo beans
- ½ cup, dried tomatoes
- ½ chopped onion
- 3 tbsp olive oil
- 1 cup chicken broth
- 2 tsp butter
- Salt, as per your taste
- ½ cup dry rice
- Parsley to garnish

1. Drain and chop sun-dried tomatoes. In a pot, sauté tomatoes, onion, and 2 tbsp olive oil.
2. Add broth and simmer it. In another pot, heat 1 tbsp olive oil and butter.
3. Add rice and sauté. Blend the sauce from the first pot and pour it over the rice.
4. Add garbanzo beans and salt and cook on low heat.
5. Cover and let sit for 15 minutes. Garnish with parsley before serving.

Balilah

VEGETARIAN, DAIRY FREE, GLUTEN FREE
PREP TIME: 05 MIN **COOK TIME:** 00 MIN **SERVINGS:** 4
Calories: 160, Carbs: 18g, Protein: 5g, Fat: 7g, Fiber: 4g, Sodium: 120mg

- 2 cups canned chickpeas, rinsed and drained
- 2 tbsp olive oil
- 2 tbsp lemon juice
- ¼ tsp ground cumin
- ¼ cup fresh parsley, chopped

1. In a large mixing bowl, add the chickpeas, olive oil, lemon juice, and ground cumin.
2. Gently toss the ingredients until the chickpeas are well-coated with the dressing.
3. Sprinkle the fresh parsley on top and mix again. Serve immediately or refrigerate for up to 2 hours for enhanced flavor.

Risotto alla Puttanesca

DAIRY FREE
PREP TIME: 05 MIN **COOK TIME:** 25 MIN **SERVINGS:** 4
Calories: 420, Carbs: 47g, Protein: 6g, Fat: 22g, Fiber: 4g, Sodium: 340mg

- 20 oz tomato puree
- 2 cup vegetable broth
- 6-8 basil leaves, divided
- 2 tsp salt
- 1 tsp pepper
- 4 tbsp olive oil
- 4 garlic cloves, crushed
- 4 anchovy fillets
- ⅔ cups grain rice
- ½ cup dry white wine
- 2 tbsp olive oil
- 1 tbsp capers
- 4 tbsp black olives, chopped

1. In a pot, dilute tomato sauce with broth and heat over low.
2. Add half the basil, pepper, and salt, and keep warm. In a pan, heat olive oil.
3. Add garlic and anchovies, melting anchovies over low heat.
4. Remove garlic and add rice. Toast rice, then deglaze with wine. Gradually add tomato sauce.
5. After 20 minutes, when rice is tender, stir in olive oil, capers, and olives. Turn off heat and cover.
6. Let it rest for 5 minutes. Serve with remaining basil.

Black Olive Tapenade With Pasta

VEGETARIAN
PREP TIME: 15 MIN **COOK TIME:** 15 MIN **SERVINGS:** 6
Calories: 537, Carbs: 59g, Protein: 13g, Fat: 28g, Fiber: 4g, Sodium: 169mg

- 2 garlic cloves
- 2 cups black olives
- ¼ cup parsley
- 1 tsp capers
- 6 anchovy fillets
- Ground pepper to taste
- Salt to taste
- ½ cup olive oil
- 1 lb spaghetti
- ¼ cup parmesan cheese
- ¼ cups black olives (pitted)

1. Blend garlic, olives, parsley, capers, anchovies, pepper, and salt. Slowly add olive oil until smooth.
2. Boil salted water and cook spaghetti as directed.
3. Drain pasta and toss with olive paste. Serve with Parmesan and extra olives.

Buckwheat Pancakes

VEGETARIAN, DAIRY FREE

PREP TIME: 10 MIN **COOK TIME:** 20 MIN **SERVINGS:** 2

Calories: 572, Carbs: 90g, Protein: 10g, Fat: 20g,
Fiber: 5g, Sodium: 144mg

- ⅔ cup buckwheat flour
- 1 tsp baking powder
- ¼ tsp baking soda
- ¼ salt
- 1 egg
- ¼ cup coconut cream
- ¾ cup almond milk
- 1 tsp vanilla
- 2 tsp maple syrup
- 4 tsp olive oil

Toppings (optional):
- ½ cup full fat yogurt
- ¼ cup maple syrup

1. Combine buckwheat flour, baking powder, baking soda, and salt in a bowl.
2. Whisk egg, coconut cream, almond milk, vanilla, and 2 tsp maple syrup in another bowl.
3. Add dry ingredients to wet and stir gently (don't overmix).
4. Heat olive oil in a skillet. Fry pancakes, flipping when bubbles form. Top with yogurt and 1 tbsp maple syrup.

White Beans with Tahini

VEGETARIAN

PREP TIME: 15 MIN **COOK TIME:** 01 MIN **SERVINGS:** 4

Calories: 514, Carbs: 52g, Protein: 19g, Fat: 28g,
Fiber: 9g, Sodium: 229mg

- ¾ cup tahini
- 1 lemon, squeezed
- 2 garlic cloves, minced
- Salt, as per taste
- ⅓ cup water
- 1 can (28 oz) white beans
- 2 pita bread, toasted and diced

For Drizzling:
- 1 tbsp olive oil
- ½ tsp red pepper flakes
- ¼ tsp cayenne
- ½ tsp cumin

For Serving:
- 3 sprigs parsley, chopped

1. Mix tahini, lemon juice, garlic, water, and salt in a bowl.
2. Stir in white beans and set aside.
3. Heat olive oil, add spices, and cook.
4. Top toasted pita with the bean mixture.
5. Drizzle with spiced olive oil and garnish with parsley. Serve.

Turkish Lentil Mezze

VEGETARIAN, DAIRY FREE

PREP TIME: 10 MIN **COOK TIME:** 20 MIN **SERVINGS:** 4

Calories: 307, Carbs: 48g, Protein: 13g, Fat: 8g,
Fiber: 16g, Sodium: 289mg

- 3 cups hot water
- 2 tbsp olive oil
- 2 onions, chopped
- 1 tbsp tomato paste
- 1 tbsp red pepper
- ¾ cup red lentils, rinsed
- ¾ cup bulgur
- 4 green onions, chopped
- 1 bunch parsley, chopped
- 1 ½ tsp cumin
- 1 tsp pepper
- Salt and pepper, to taste

1. Boil water. Cook onions in olive oil. Add tomato and red pepper paste, mix, and cool.
2. Simmer rinsed lentils in water. Drain excess liquid and cool.
3. Stir bulgur with hot water. Cover and let it absorb. In a bowl, mix lentils, bulgur, sautéed onions, green onions, parsley, cumin, salt, and pepper.
4. Wet hands with olive oil and knead mixture into a soft dough.
5. Form into ovals and place on a plate with lettuce. Serve with lemon or pomegranate molasses.

Tuna Pasta with Peas

DAIRY FREE

PREP TIME: 05 MIN **COOK TIME:** 15 MIN **SERVINGS:** 2

Calories: 538, Carbs: 74g, Protein: 38g, Fat: 16g,
Fiber: 6g, Sodium: 442mg

- 6 oz penne pasta
- 1 tbsp olive oil
- 2 garlic cloves, minced
- 1 can (5 oz) albacore tuna in oil
- ½ cup peas, frozen or fresh
- ⅓ cup tomato puree
- Salt and pepper, to taste

1. Boil salted water, cook penne al dente.
2. Heat olive oil, cook tuna and garlic for 2-3 minutes.
3. Add peas, cook for 2 minutes.
4. Stir in tomato purée, season, cook 10 minutes.
5. Drain pasta, toss with sauce for 30 seconds.
6. Serve.

Sicilian Almond Pasta

VEGETARIAN

PREP TIME: 10 MIN **COOK TIME:** 20 MIN **SERVINGS:** 4

Calories: 350, Carbs: 55g, Protein: 10g, Fat: 10g, Fiber: 6g, Sodium: 301mg

- Kosher salt, to taste
- 10 cherry tomatoes
- ½ cup almonds
- 1 cup basil leaves
- ¾ cup mint leaves
- 1 handful chopped arugula
- 1 chopped garlic clove
- Ground black pepper
- ½ cup olive oil
- ½ cup cheese (Pecorino Romano)
- 1 lb spiral shaped pasta, for serving (optional)

1. Heat oven to 375°F. Boil salted water for pasta. Score tomatoes, blanch 1 minute, peel.
2. Blanch and toast almonds. Blend tomatoes, almonds, herbs, garlic, salt, and pepper.
3. Add olive oil, then stir in Pecorino. Cook pasta until al dente. Reserve 1 cup pasta water, drain.
4. Toss pasta with pesto, adding pasta water to loosen.
5. Plate pasta, top with extra pesto and Pecorino.

Spanish Rice and Beans

VEGETARIAN, DAIRY FREE

PREP TIME: 05 MIN **COOK TIME:** 25 MIN **SERVINGS:** 4

Calories: 487, Carbs: 90g, Protein: 18g, Fat: 6g, Fiber: 12g, Sodium: 124mg

- 2 tbsp olive oil
- 1 onion, chopped
- Kosher salt, as per taste
- 2 garlic cloves, minced
- 1 tsp sweet paprika
- 1 tsp ground cumin
- ½ tsp red pepper flakes (optional)
- 2 cups basmati rice, rinsed
- 2 cans (15 oz each) kidney beans,
- 1 can (15 oz) diced fire roasted tomatoes
- 2 tbsp tomato paste
- 2 ½ cup vegetable broth
- ⅓ cup green olives, sliced (optional)
- ¼ cup cilantro, chopped (optional)

1. Heat olive oil in a pan. Cook onion until softened.
2. Add salt to it. Stir in garlic, paprika, cumin, and red pepper flakes. Cook for 30 seconds.
3. Stir in rice, salt, beans, and tomatoes. Mix tomato paste with broth, then add to pan.
4. Bring to a boil, reduce to low, cover, and simmer till rice is cooked.
5. Garnish with olives and parsley, then serve.

Creamy Orzo with Garlic, Parmesan and Blistered Tomatoes

VEGETARIAN

PREP TIME: 05 MIN **COOK TIME:** 20 MIN **SERVINGS:** 4

Calories: 369, Carbs: 54g, Protein: 18g, Fat: 4g, Fiber: 6g, Sodium: 234mg

- 2 tbsp olive oil
- 4 garlic cloves, chopped
- Salt, to taste
- 5 cups tomatoes
- 2 cups dry orzo
- 4 cups broth
- 1 cup yogurt
- ¼ cup parmesan, grated

1. Heat oil in a pan, add tomatoes, garlic, salt, and pepper. Cover and cook.
2. Mash tomatoes and cook uncovered until juicy.
3. Add orzo, cover with broth/water, season, and cook, stirring occasionally.
4. Mix warm broth with yogurt to bring it to room temp. Stir yogurt into pasta, add cheese, adjust seasoning, and serve.

Butter Beans with Garlic, Lemon & Herbs

VEGETARIAN, GLUTEN FREE

PREP TIME: 05 MIN **COOK TIME:** 07 MIN **SERVINGS:** 4

Calories: 245, Carbs: 34g, Protein: 11g, Fat: 7g, Fiber: 10g, Sodium: 221mg

- 2 tsp olive oil
- ½ tsp red pepper flakes
- ½ tsp Urfa pepper (optional)
- ½ tsp cumin
- ¼ tsp smoked paprika
- 4 garlic cloves, minced
- Kosher salt, as per taste
- Black pepper, as per taste
- 2 cans butter beans (30oz)
- 2 lemons, juiced
- 2 green onions, chopped
- ⅓ cup chopped parsley
- ⅓ cup chopped dill

1. Heat olive oil, add spices and garlic. Stir for 30 seconds.
2. Add beans and broth, boil, then simmer for 5-10 minutes. Stir in lemon juice, green onions, and herbs.
3. Serve with bread, rice, or pasta.

Toasted Orzo with Parmesan and Sundried Tomatoes

VEGETARIAN

PREP TIME: 05 MIN **COOK TIME:** 10 MIN **SERVINGS:** 4

Calories: 547, Carbs: 50g, Protein: 13g, Fat: 33g, Fiber: 4g, Sodium: 174mg

- 2 tbsp olive oil
- 1 ½ cups orzo pasta
- 7 cups boiling water
- ½ cup olive oil
- 5 garlic cloves, minced
- ½ lemon
- ¾ cups parmesan, grated
- 1 cup parsley
- ½ cup dill
- ⅓ cup dried tomatoes, chopped
- Salt and pepper, to taste

1. Heat olive oil in a saucepan over medium-high. Toast orzo until golden.
2. Add boiling water and salt. Cook orzo. Reserve 1 cup water, then drain.
3. Heat ½ cup olive oil. Add garlic, salt, and red pepper flakes.
4. Cook until fragrant. Stir in lemon juice, pasta water, parsley, dill.
5. Add pasta to sauce, toss with sundried tomatoes and Parmesan.
6. Add more pasta water if needed. Top with extra Parmesan and red pepper flakes.

Lebanese Rice with Vermicelli

VEGETARIAN, DAIRY FREE

PREP TIME: 05 MIN **COOK TIME:** 20 MIN **SERVINGS:** 4

Calories: 331, Carbs: 61g, Protein: 6g, Fat: 5g, Fiber: 2g, Sodium: 211mg

- 2 cups long grain rice
- Water
- 1 cup broken vermicelli
- 2 ½ tbsp olive oil
- Salt, as per taste
- ½ cup toasted pine nuts (optional)

1. Rinse rice, soak, then drain. Heat olive oil, toast vermicelli until golden.
2. Add rice, salt, 3 ½ cups water. Boil until water reduces by half.
3. Cover, cook on low heat. Let sit, then fluff. Top with pine nuts.

Farro Risotto

VEGETARIAN

PREP TIME: 10 MIN **COOK TIME:** 20 MIN **SERVINGS:** 4

Calories: 366, Carbs: 54g, Protein: 16g, Fat: 12g, Fiber: 6g, Sodium: 621mg

- 2 tbsp olive oil
- 3 green onions, chopped
- 8 oz Bella mushrooms
- 1 cup frozen peas
- 1 tsp chopped garlic
- 1 cup Italian farro
- 1 tsp sweet paprika
- Salt and pepper, to taste
- 2 ¼ cup vegetable broth
- ½ cup parmesan cheese
- ¼ cup mint leaves

1. Heat olive oil in a skillet over medium-high. Sauté green onions, mushrooms, and peas.
2. Add garlic, cook 30 seconds. Stir in farro, paprika, salt, and pepper. Cook for 4-5 minutes.
3. Add boiling broth, bring to a boil. Reduce heat, cover, and simmer.
4. Remove from heat, stir in Parmesan and mint. Serve warm.

Garlic Parmesan White Beans

VEGETARIAN, GLUTEN FREE

PREP TIME: 10 MIN **COOK TIME:** 15 MIN **SERVINGS:** 4

Calories: 316, Carbs: 50g, Protein: 21g, Fat: 4g, Fiber: 11g, Sodium: 549mg

- 4 garlic cloves, minced
- 2 tbsp olive oil
- 2 cans (30oz) cannellini beans
- ½ cup water
- Salt and pepper, to taste
- 1 tsp Aleppo pepper
- ½ tsp cumin
- 1 cup cherry tomatoes, halved
- 1 cup parsley, chopped
- ¼ cup parmesan, shaved
- ¼ cup Pecorino Romano, grated
- Half lemon, juiced

1. Heat olive oil in a pan. Add garlic and cook until golden.
2. Add cannellini beans, ½ cup water, salt, pepper, spices, and tomatoes. Cook for 10 minutes, stirring occasionally.
3. Stir in parsley, cheese, and lemon juice.
4. Drizzle with olive oil and serve with pita or bread.

CHAPTER 9
FISH & SEAFOOD

Get ready to dive into the Mediterranean's ocean of flavors! From sizzling grilled fish to juicy shrimp and mouthwatering seafood stews, this chapter is all about celebrating the freshest catches. Simple ingredients, bold flavors, and the taste of the sea—these dishes will transport you straight to the coast. Let's reel in some deliciousness!

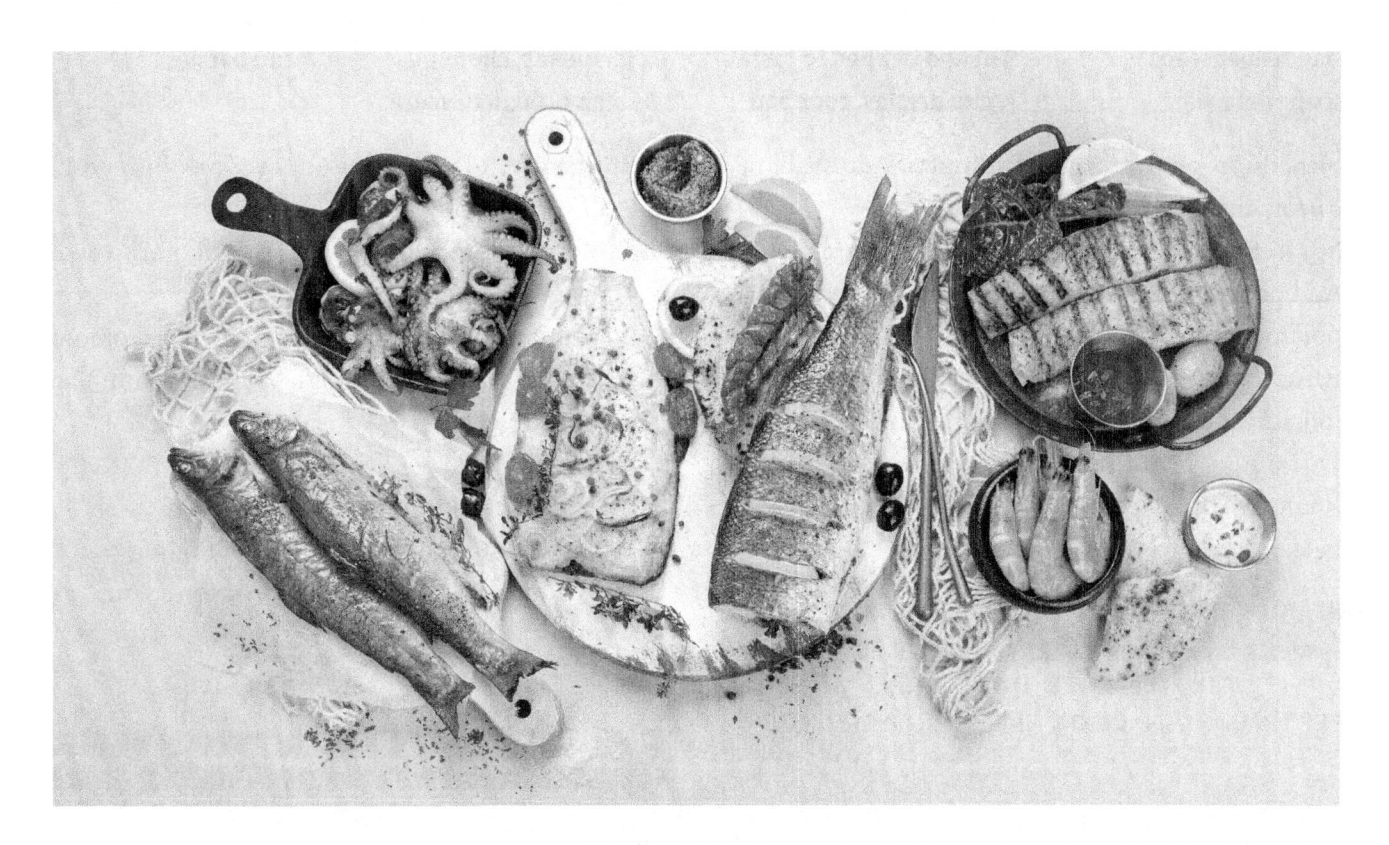

TIPS

- Always opt for fresh, sustainably sourced seafood for the best flavor and texture.

- Let the natural flavors of seafood shine with just olive oil, lemon, garlic, and herbs.

- Seafood cooks quickly—be mindful to avoid overcooking to keep it tender and juicy.

Mussels with Chorizo

GLUTEN FREE, DAIRY FREE
PREP TIME: 10 MIN **COOK TIME:** 20 MIN **SERVINGS:** 4
Calories: 260, Carbs: 20g, Protein: 16g, Fat: 11g, Fiber: 3g, Sodium: 385mg

- 1 tbsp olive oil
- 3 oz smoked chorizo
- 1 shallot, diced
- 1 carrot, diced
- 2 garlic cloves, minced
- ½ tsp fennel seeds
- ½ cup white wine
- ½ lb red small potatoes, cut into pieces
- 14.5 oz canned tomatoes
- 2 cups water
- 1 ½ lb mussels
- Salt and pepper, to taste
- ¼ cup parsley, chopped

1. Heat oil, cook chorizo for 5 minutes. Add shallot, carrot, and garlic; cook until soft.
2. Stir in fennel, and wine; cook until wine evaporates. Add potatoes, tomatoes, and water; simmer until potatoes are tender.
3. Rinse and remove beards from mussels. Add mussels, cover, and cook until open.
4. Discard unopened mussels.
5. Remove half the mussels, discard shells, and stir back into chowder. Season and serve.

Grilled Oysters

GLUTEN FREE, DAIRY FREE
PREP TIME: 15 MIN **COOK TIME:** 5 MIN **SERVINGS:** 4
Calories: 68, Carbs: 1g, Protein: 1g, Fat: 7g, Fiber: 1g, Sodium: 156mg

- 2 tbsp olive oil
- 2 garlic cloves, minced
- ¼ tsp Aleppo pepper
- 1 tsp fresh lemon juice
- ¼ tbsp salt
- Ground pepper to taste
- 1 tbsp parsley, minced
- 3-4 cups rock salt
- 12 live oysters, shucked

1. Heat oil, sauté garlic and Aleppo pepper for 30 seconds.
2. Stir in lemon juice, salt, pepper, and herbs. Heat oven to 400-500°F. Place oysters in rock salt, top with sauce.
3. Cook on the grill until the edges curl.
4. Serve oysters directly or transfer to a platter with rock salt.

Spicy Couscous Recipe with Shrimp

GLUTEN FREE, DAIRY FREE
PREP TIME: 15 MIN **COOK TIME:** 20 MIN **SERVINGS:** 6
Calories: 332, Carbs: 32g, Protein: 33g, Fat: 8g, Fiber: 3g, Sodium: 179mg

- 2 ½ cups water
- 6 oz chicken, cubed
- 1 tbsp olive oil
- 1 yellow onion, sliced
- 3 garlic cloves, chopped
- 2 jalapenos, chopped
- 1 ¼ tsp ground turmeric
- 1 ¼ tsp paprika
- 1 ¼ tsp ground cumin
- Salt, to taste
- 1 ½ lb shrimp
- 1 ¼ cup couscous
- 1 cup parsley

1. Bring water to a boil in a pot over medium heat.
2. Heat olive oil in a pot.
3. Add chicken and cook until crispy and browned. Transfer to paper towels to drain.
4. Add onion, garlic, and jalapeno. Stir until onions are translucent. Add turmeric, paprika, cumin and salt. Stir to coat.
5. Add shrimp and cook until pink and firm. Return cooked chicken to the pot.
6. Stir in couscous, olive oil, salt, and boiling water. Turn off the heat, cover, and let sit until couscous absorbs the liquid.
7. Uncover, stir in parsley, and serve.

Spanish Seafood Pasta

DAIRY FREE
PREP TIME: 10 MIN **COOK TIME:** 20 MIN **SERVINGS:** 4
Calories: 232, Carbs: 13g, Protein: 18g, Fat: 10g, Fiber: 3g, Sodium: 642mg

- 3 ½ cups fish broth
- 3 tbsp olive oil
- 14 oz vermicelli noodles
- 12 shrimp
- 1 onion, chopped
- ½ lb squid fresh, chopped into pieces
- 4 garlic cloves, thinly sliced
- 1 cup canned crushed tomatoes
- 1 tsp smoked paprika
- 1 tsp salt
- 1 cup dry white wine
- ½ lb mussels
- 3 tbsp flat leaf parsley
- 1 lemon

1. Simmer broth on low heat. Toast vermicelli in oil. Set it aside. Sear shrimp in oil. Set it aside.

2. Sauté onion in oil for 5 minutes. Add squid and cook. Add garlic, tomato, paprika, and salt.
3. Cook for 2 minutes. Stir in wine, reduce for 1 minute. Add vermicelli, pour in stock, and simmer.
4. Add mussels and shrimp. Cook until pasta absorbs broth, about 10 minutes.
5. Let sit, discard unopened mussels. Garnish with parsley, serve with lemon and aioli.

Tuna Rillettes

GLUTEN FREE

PREP TIME: 10 MIN COOK TIME: 10 MIN SERVINGS: 2
Calories: 149, Carbs: 3g, Protein: 15g, Fat: 13g, Fiber: 1g, Sodium: 585mg

- 5-7 oz wild caught tuna
- 1 shallot, chopped
- 2 tbsp chives
- 1 tbsp sour cream
- 1 tbsp cream cheese
- 2 tbsp heavy cream
- ½ tbsp olive oil
- ½ tsp mustard
- Salt and pepper, to taste

1. Drain and mash the tuna. Mix with the remaining ingredients.
2. Season with salt and pepper. Serve with crackers, bread, or veggies.

Moroccan Fish Kofta

GLUTEN FREE

PREP TIME: 10 MIN COOK TIME: 15 MIN SERVINGS: 4
Calories: 243, Carbs: 25g, Protein: 26g, Fat: 6g, Fiber: 4g, Sodium: 236mg

- 2 tbsp olive oil
- 3 garlic cloves, minced
- 15 oz diced tomatoes
- 1 cup vegetable broth
- 2 tbsp harissa paste
- ½ cup chopped cilantro
- ½ tsp ras el hanout
- ½ tsp cumin
- ½ lemon
- Salt, a pinch
- Black pepper, to taste

For Fish Kofta:
- 1 lb White fish fillet, cut into large pieces
- 1 onion, quartered
- 2 garlic cloves, chopped
- ½ cup fresh cilantro
- ½ cup fresh parsley
- 1 hot chili pepper, stemmed (optional)
- 1 tsp ras el hanout
- ½ tsp ground ginger
- ½ tbsp ground cinnamon
- Salt and pepper, to taste
- ½ cup dried breadcrumbs
- ½ tbsp olive oil
- 1 egg

1. Heat olive oil, cook garlic 30 seconds.
2. Add tomatoes, broth, harissa, peppers, cilantro, spices, lemon, salt, and pepper. Simmer, covered with a small opening.
3. Blend fish, onion, garlic, cilantro, parsley, chili (optional), and rase el hanout, ginger, and cinnamon in a food processor.
4. Add salt, pepper, and pulse. Mix in breadcrumbs, egg, and olive oil. Shape into 1-tbsp balls.
5. Place in sauce, cover partially, and cook for 10-15 minutes. Garnish with cilantro/parsley.

Linguine with Clams

GLUTEN FREE, DAIRY FREE

PREP TIME: 15 MIN COOK TIME: 15 MIN SERVINGS: 4
Calories: 424, Carbs: 58g, Protein: 14g, Fat: 13g, Fiber: 3g, Sodium: 631mg

- 2 lb littleneck clams
- ⅓ cup olive oil
- 1 garlic clove, minced
- ½ cup dry white wine
- 1 lb linguine
- 2 tbsp leaf parsley, chopped

1. Scrub and soak clams in salted water. Drain and rinse.
2. To boil pasta add water and salt in a pan and bring it to a boil.
3. Cook clams with 2 tbsp water in a covered skillet over medium-high heat until open. Discard any that don't open. Let cool.
4. Set aside 3-4 whole clams per serving. Remove meat from remaining clams and set aside.
5. Strain remaining liquid through a fine sieve into a bowl.
6. Sauté garlic and red pepper flakes in olive oil over medium-low heat for 5 minutes. Add wine, simmer for 1 minute, then stir in clam juice and meat. Heat through for 2-3 minutes.
7. Boil pasta 1-2 minutes less than package directions.
8. Toss pasta in sauce over low heat, adding pasta water if needed.
9. Stir in parsley and top with reserved clams. Serve immediately

Spaghetti with Garlicky Sautéed Shrimp

DAIRY FREE

PREP TIME: 10 MIN **COOK TIME:** 20 MIN **SERVINGS:** 4

Calories: 462, Carbs: 58g, Protein: 24g, Fat: 13g, Fiber: 3g, Sodium: 184mg

- 2 tsp salt
- 1 tbsp black peppercorns
- 3 tbsp olive oil
- 1 garlic clove, minced
- 3 tbsp dry white wine
- 2 tbsp lemon juice
- 18-24 large shrimp
- 1 lb spaghetti
- 4 oz Pecorino

1. Bring salted water to a boil and cook pasta.
2. Reserve 1 ½ cups pasta water, then drain.
3. Toast peppercorns in a skillet until aromatic, then grind coarsely. Sauté garlic in olive oil, add wine, lemon juice, zest, and shrimp.
4. Cook until shrimp is opaque. Remove shrimp, increase heat to thicken sauce for 30-60 seconds.
5. Cover to keep warm. Toss pasta in the sauce with reserved pasta water, cheese, and crushed pepper.
6. Stir until creamy, adding more water if needed.
7. Plate pasta, top with shrimp, remaining cheese, pepper, and parsley. Serve immediately.

Egyptian Fried Fish Sandwich

DAIRY FREE

PREP TIME: 10 MIN **COOK TIME:** 20 MIN **SERVINGS:** 4

Calories: 308, Carbs: 49g, Protein: 27g, Fat: 2g, Fiber: 7g, Sodium: 156mg

- 1½ lb fish fillet, sliced into 4 pieces
- 1 tsp ground coriander
- 1 tsp ground cumin
- 1 tbsp paprika
- ½ tsp Aleppo pepper
- Salt, a pinch
- Pepper, a pinch
- 3 garlic cloves, minced
- 3 lemons, halved
- Oil for frying
- 1 cup all-purpose flour
- ½ cup cornstarch
- 1 tsp baking soda
- **To serve (optional):**
- Tahini sauce
- 1 large tomato, diced
- 2 Persian cucumber, diced
- 2 cups baby arugula, diced
- Pita bread, halved
- Olives, pitted

1. Pat fish dry, coat with spice mix and garlic, squeeze lemon juice over it, and refrigerate.
2. Slice cucumber, tomato, pickles. Smash and pit olives if using.
3. Coat fillets with flour, cornstarch, and baking soda mixture.
4. Heat oil and fry fish 3 minutes per side until golden. Drain on paper towels and squeeze lemon juice over.
5. Spread tahini sauce in pita, add veggies, fish, and more tahini sauce. Serve with olives and pickles.

Tunisian Salad

DAIRY FREE

PREP TIME: 10 MIN **COOK TIME:** 20 MIN **SERVINGS:** 4

Calories: 298, Carbs: 17g, Protein: 16g, Fat: 20g, Fiber: 5g, Sodium: 234mg

- 4 tbsp olive oil
- 1 ½ tbsp white wine vinegar
- 1 tsp parsley
- ¾ tsp black pepper
- ¾ tsp salt
- ½ lemon juiced
- 8 Roma tomatoes, diced
- 1 apple, diced
- 1 red onion, diced
- Handful mint leaves, chopped
- 5 hard-boiled eggs
- ½ cup black & green olives
- 5 oz canned tuna

1. Shake olive oil, vinegar, parsley, salt, pepper, and lemon juice in a jar (or whisk in a bowl).
2. Dice tomatoes, and apple. Combine tomatoes, apple, and mint in a bowl.
3. Add dressing you made earlier and toss. Stir in onion, adjust to taste.
4. Top with egg wedges, olives, and tuna. Serve with baguette slices.

Mussels Marinara with Fennel (Greece)

GLUTEN FREE

PREP TIME: 10 MIN **COOK TIME:** 20 MIN **SERVINGS:** 6

Calories: 310, Carbs: 16g, Protein: 19g, Fat: 16g, Fiber: 4g, Sodium: 189mg

- 3 lb fresh live mussels in the shell
- 1 cup white wine
- 2 garlic cloves, minced
- ½ bunch fresh parsley
- 1 onion, chopped
- 2 tbsp fresh oregano, chopped

- 2 tsp sage, chopped
- 2 tbsp fennel seeds
- ¼ cup olive oil
- 8 oz tomato sauce
- 1 tbsp tomato paste
- 1 dash cayenne pepper
- ½ tsp paprika
- 4 oz feta cheese
- Sea salt, to taste

1. Discard open mussels. Cook mussels, white wine, garlic, and parsley in a pot. Remove from heat, keep covered.
2. Dice vegetables and crush fennel seeds.
3. Take mussels out of shells, discard shells and parsley stalks. Reserve broth.
4. Sauté onion in oil until browned. Add pepper and fennel, cook 5 minutes. Add sage, cook 2-3 minutes.
5. Add mussels and oregano, cook 1-2 minutes. Stir in tomato sauce, paste, and mussel broth. Add hot pepper and paprika, simmer.
6. Remove from heat, cool 2-3 minutes. Add feta and parsley. Serve.

Greek Fish with Onions and Tomatoes

DAIRY FREE, GLUTEN FREE
PREP TIME: 10 MIN **COOK TIME:** 20 MIN **SERVINGS:** 4
Calories: 160, Carbs: 10g, Protein: 29g, Fat: 2g, Fiber: 3g, Sodium: 269mg

- 2 tbsp olive oil
- 1 onion, chopped
- 2 garlic cloves, mined
- 28 oz peeled tomatoes
- 2 tsp dried oregano
- 2 lb halibut fish filet
- 1 tsp sweet paprika
- ½ tsp ground cumin
- 2 lemons
- ¼ cup parsley
- Salt and pepper, to taste

1. Preheat oven to 400°F. Sauté onions in olive oil with salt until golden (7 min).
2. Add garlic, tomatoes, salt, oregano, and pepper. Simmer for 10-15 minutes.
3. Pat dry the fish, season with salt, oregano, paprika, cumin, and squeeze 1 lemon over.
4. Place fish in sauce, spoon sauce over. Bake until fish flakes.
5. Garnish with parsley and lemon wedges.

Seafood Paella

GLUTEN FREE, DAIRY FREE
PREP TIME: 10 MIN **COOK TIME:** 20 MIN **SERVINGS:** 4
Calories: 210, Carbs: 31g, Protein: 14g, Fat: 3g, Fiber: 2g, Sodium: 300mg

- 1 cup arborio rice
- 2 cups chicken broth
- ½ lb shrimp, peeled and deveined
- ½ cup frozen peas
- ¼ tsp smoked paprika

1. In a large skillet, bring the chicken broth to a boil over medium heat. Add the arborio rice and reduce the heat to low. Cover and cook for 15 minutes, stirring occasionally.
2. Stir in the shrimp, frozen peas, and smoked paprika. Cover and cook for another 5 minutes, or until the shrimp are pink and cooked through.
3. Remove the skillet from heat, fluff the rice with a fork, and serve immediately.

Mediterranean Salmon Kabobs

GLUTEN FREE, DAIRY FREE
PREP TIME: 10 MIN **COOK TIME:** 20 MIN **SERVINGS:** 4
Calories: 479, Carbs: 18g, Protein: 40g, Fat: 28g, Fiber: 13g, Sodium: 376mg

- 1.5 lb salmon fillet, cubes
- 1 zucchini, round slices
- 1 onion, cut into squares
- Salt, as per taste
- ¼ cup olive oil
- 1 juiced lemon
- 3 garlic cloves, minced
- 2 tsp fresh thyme leaves
- 2 tsp dry oregano
- 1 tsp ground cumin
- 1 tsp chili pepper
- ½ tsp ground coriander

1. Whisk olive oil, lemon juice, garlic, oregano, thyme, cumin, chili pepper, and coriander for marinade.
2. Toss salmon, zucchini, and onions with marinade. Let sit for 15-20 minutes.
3. Thread salmon, zucchini, and onions onto skewers. Heat olive oil in a skillet over medium heat.
4. Cook skewers for 6-8 minutes, turning halfway, until salmon is cooked through. Serve.

Cod with Tomato Sauce

GLUTEN FREE, DAIRY FREE

PREP TIME: 5 MIN **COOK TIME:** 25 MIN **SERVINGS:** 4

Calories: 293, Carbs: 22g, Protein: 34g, Fat: 9g, Fiber: 4g, Sodium: 544mg

- 1 onion, chopped
- 2 garlic, chopped
- 2 tbsp olive oil
- 3 cups tomato puree
- 1 tsp sugar
- ½ tsp, salt
- 8 medium loins of desalted cod
- 2 roasted red peppers

1. Chop garlic and onion. Heat oil in a pan, sauté garlic and onion until golden.
2. Add tomato puree, sugar, and salt. Simmer for 15 minutes.
3. Add the cod fillets to the simmering sauce. Cook for 6-8 minutes per side, or until the fish is opaque.
4. Add chopped peppers, cook for a few more minutes and serve. (Add broth or water if needed).

Shrimp Fra Diavolo

GLUTEN FREE, DAIRY FREE

PREP TIME: 10 MIN **COOK TIME:** 20 MIN **SERVINGS:** 4

Calories: 194, Carbs: 17g, Protein: 18g, Fat: 2g, Fiber: 3g, Sodium: 329mg

- 1 lb shrimp
- Salt, to taste
- 2 tsp red pepper flakes
- Olive oil, to taste
- 1 onion, chopped
- 5 garlic cloves, minced
- 1 cup white wine
- 15 oz diced fire roasted tomatoes
- ¼ cup tomato paste
- 2 tsp dried oregano
- ½ cup chopped fresh parsley

1. Pat shrimp dry, season with salt and red pepper flakes.
2. Heat 2 tbsp olive oil in a skillet, cook shrimp 45 seconds to 1 minute, transfer to a plate. In same skillet, heat olive oil.
3. Sauté onions and garlic. Add white wine and cook until reduced by half.
4. Stir in tomatoes, tomato paste, salt, pepper, oregano, and red pepper flakes. Simmer.
5. Return shrimp to the skillet, cook for 1 minute until pink.
6. Garnish with parsley and serve with bread, pasta, or rice.

Lemony Shrimp Risotto

GLUTEN FREE

PREP TIME: 10 MIN **COOK TIME:** 20 MIN **SERVINGS:** 4

Calories: 523, Carbs: 67g, Protein: 27g, Fat: 17g, Fiber: 4g, Sodium: 221mg

- 3 tbsp olive oil
- 1 lb large shrimp
- 1 tsp salt
- 1 lemon, zest
- ⅛ tsp red pepper, crushed
- ¼ cup shallot, chopped
- 1 ½ cup glute free arborio rice
- 4 cups vegetable broth
- 4 cups torn spinach leaves
- 1 tbsp unsalted butter

1. Sauté shrimp in 1 tbsp olive oil with ¼ tsp salt for 3-4 minutes.
2. Set aside and toss with lemon zest and red pepper flakes. Sauté shallots in 2 tbsp olive oil for 2-3 minutes.
3. Add rice and cook. Add broth and ½ tsp salt. Cover and cook until rice is tender.
4. Stir in spinach, butter, and remaining salt until spinach wilts. Top with shrimp and their juice.

Fish en Papillote, Mediterranean-style

GLUTEN FREE, DAIRY FREE

PREP TIME: 10 MIN **COOK TIME:** 15 MIN **SERVINGS:** 4

Calories: 222, Carbs: 5g, Protein: 27g, Fat: 12g, Fiber: 2g, Sodium: 188mg

- 1 ¼ lb cod fish fillet
- Salt, a pinch
- ½ tomato, thinly sliced
- ½ green bell pepper, thinly sliced into 4 rounds
- ½ lemon, sliced into rings
- ¼ cup olive oil
- ½ lemon, juiced
- 1 shallot, chopped
- 2 garlic cloves, chopped
- 1 tsp oregano
- 1 tsp paprika
- ½ tsp cumin

1. Preheat oven to 425°F. Season fish with salt and pepper.
2. Whisk olive oil, lemon juice, shallots, garlic, and spices. Cut 4 large pieces of parchment paper (12 inches), fold in half.
3. Place fish on parchment, spoon sauce, top with lemon, tomato, and bell pepper.

4. Seal pouches and bake on a sheet for 12-15 minutes, until fish flakes. Serve in parchment pouches.

Za'atar Garlic Salmon

GLUTEN FREE, DAIRY FREE

PREP TIME: 10 MIN **COOK TIME:** 25 MIN **SERVINGS:** 4

Calories: 332, Carbs: 29g, Protein: 24g, Fat: 14g, Fiber: 8g, Sodium: 539mg

- 12 potatoes, scrubbed
- 2 cups grape tomatoes, halved
- 6 oz broccoli florets
- 3 tbsp fresh minced garlic
- Salt and pepper, to taste
- Olive oil
- 2 tsp za'atar spice
- 1 tsp coriander
- 1 lb salmon fillet
- 1 lemon, juiced

1. Preheat oven to 400°F. Toss vegetables (potatoes, tomatoes, broccoli) with 2 tbsp olive oil, salt, pepper, garlic, za'atar, and coriander.
2. Spread on a baking sheet. Season salmon with salt, pepper, olive oil, garlic, za'atar, and coriander.
3. Place salmon on the sheet with vegetables. Drizzle with more olive oil if needed.
4. Bake the salmon. Finish with lemon juice and more za'atar. Serve with rice and salad.

Lemon Garlic Shrimp with Peas and Artichokes

GLUTEN FREE

PREP TIME: 05 MIN **COOK TIME:** 15 MIN **SERVINGS:** 4

Calories: 240, Carbs: 13g, Protein: 27g, Fat: 10g, Fiber: 6g, Sodium: 358mg

- 1 ½ tsp ground coriander
- 1 tsp Aleppo pepper
- 1 tsp sweet paprika
- 1 lb large shrimps
- Salt and pepper, to taste
- 1 onion, sliced
- 8 garlic cloves, chopped
- 1 cup dry white wine
- 2 tbsp fresh lemon juice
- 2 tsp honey
- ½ cup chicken broth
- 1 ½ cup frozen peas
- 15 oz baby artichokes
- Parmesan, to taste
- Parsley, to taste

1. Mix coriander, Aleppo pepper and paprika (for shrimp). Season shrimp with salt, pepper, and 2 ½ tsp of spice mix. Set it aside.
2. Heat 2 tbsp olive oil in a large skillet over medium heat.
3. Add onions and cook for 5 minutes. Add garlic and cook until fragrant (do not brown).
4. Pour in white wine, cook until reduced by half. Add lemon juice, honey, and broth, bring to a boil.
5. Stir in peas, artichokes, salt, pepper, and remaining spice mix.
6. Cook for 10 minutes. Add shrimp and cook until pink, about 2-3 minutes. Remove from heat. Garnish with Parmesan and fresh parsley.
7. Serve with orzo or Lebanese rice.

Mediterranean Lemon Poached Halibut

DAIRY FREE, GLUTEN FREE

PREP TIME: 05 MIN **COOK TIME:** 25 MIN **SERVINGS:** 6

Calories: 338, Carbs: 5g, Protein: 37g, Fat: 13g, Fiber: 13g, Sodium: 684mg

For spice rub:
- 1 tsp dried oregano
- 1 tsp coriander
- ½ tsp ground paprika
- ½ tsp salt and pepper, each

For Halibut:
- 2 lb halibut fillet
- Olive oil
- ½ cup red onion, chopped
- 8 garlic cloves, minced
- 2 ½ cup chicken broth
- ½ cup white wine
- 2 large lemons, juiced and zest
- ½ cup fresh parsley, chopped
- 1 tbsp capers
- 3 scallions, chopped
- ¼ cup grated carrots

1. In a bowl, mix spices for spice rub, salt, and pepper.
2. Pat fillet dry and rub with spice blend.
3. Heat olive oil in a skillet. Add onions and cook until translucent. Add garlic and cook for 30 seconds.
4. Pour in chicken broth, wine, lemon juice, zest, parsley, and capers. Bring to a simmer, then reduce heat to low.
5. Carefully add fish, cover loosely, and cook until opaque and flaky.
6. Remove from heat, top with herbs, capers, grated carrots, and scallions.

Mediterranean Oven Roasted Spanish Mackerel

DAIRY FREE, GLUTEN FREE
PREP TIME: 05 MIN **COOK TIME:** 25 MIN **SERVINGS:** 2
Calories: 239, Carbs: 4g, Protein: 32g, Fat: 10g, Fiber: 3g, Sodium: 197mg

- 3 garlic cloves
- 1 tsp salt
- 1 tsp ground coriander
- ½ tsp ground cumin
- ¼ cup fresh parsley, chopped
- ¼ cup fresh dill
- 1 ½ lb Spanish mackerel
- 1 lemon
- 2-3 tbsp fresh lemon juice

1. Preheat oven to 350°F and warm a sheet pan.
2. Crush garlic with salt, then mix in coriander, cumin, parsley, and dill.
3. Pat fish dry, remove dark veins, and salt inside and out. Stuff fish with lemon slices and herb mixture, drizzle with olive oil.
4. Wrap fish in foil, seal, and place on sheet pan.
5. Bake for 25 minutes. Add lemon juice and serve.

Mediterranean-Style Whole Roasted Red Snapper

GLUTEN FREE, DAIRY FREE
PREP TIME: 10 MIN **COOK TIME:** 15 MIN **SERVINGS:** 6
Calories: 344, Carbs: 6g, Protein: 46g, Fat: 9g, Fiber: 4g, Sodium: 535mg

- 2 snapper fish,
- 10 garlic cloves, minced
- 2 tsp ground cumin
- 2 tsp ground coriander
- 1 tsp black pepper
- 1 tsp ground sumac
- ½ cup fresh dill
- 3 bell peppers, round slices
- 1 large tomato, round slices
- 1 onion, round slices
- 2 lemons

1. Preheat oven to 425°F.
2. Pat snapper dry. Make two slits on each side and fill with minced garlic.
3. Combine cumin, coriander, salt, pepper, and sumac. Coat the fish with 3/4 of the mix, pressing it into the slits.
4. Fill the gut cavity with dill, peppers, tomatoes, and onions.
5. Place fish on a lightly oiled sheet. Add remaining sliced vegetables around the fish, sprinkle with salt and remaining spice mix.
6. Drizzle everything with olive oil and roast on the lower rack until fish flakes.
7. Transfer fish to a platter, squeeze lemon juice over, and portion using the slits.

Steamed Mussels in Garlic White Wine Broth

GLUTEN FREE, DAIRY FREE
PREP TIME: 10 MIN **COOK TIME:** 20 MIN **SERVINGS:** 4
Calories: 332, Carbs: 14g, Protein: 41g, Fat: 11g, Fiber: 6g, Sodium: 528mg

- 4 garlic cloves, minced
- 1 large shallot, thinly sliced
- 1 tsp Italian seasoning
- ½ red pepper flakes
- 3 lb mussels
- 1 cup chicken broth
- ½ cup dry white wine
- 3 tbsp fresh parsley
- 1 lemon
- 1 French baguette (optional)

1. Rinse mussels, discarding any that don't close when tapped. Heat 2-3 tbsp olive oil in a pot.
2. Add garlic, shallots, salt, seasoning, and red pepper flakes. Cook until fragrant.
3. Add mussels, broth, and wine. Cover and steam for 5-6 minutes until mussels open.
4. Stir in parsley. Serve with lemon wedges and bread.

Stuffed Tomatoes with Tuna

DAIRY FREE, GLUTEN FREE
PREP TIME: 05 MIN **COOK TIME:** 20 MIN **SERVINGS:** 4
Calories: 143, Carbs: 9g, Protein: 16g, Fat: 6g, Fiber: 3g, Sodium: 484mg

- 1 tbsp olive oil
- 4 large tomatoes
- 1 tsp salt
- 1 onion, chopped
- 2 garlic cloves, minced
- 5 oz tuna packed
- ¼ cup chopped green olives
- 2 tbsp fresh parsley, chopped
- 1 tbsp lemon juice
- Black pepper, to taste

1. Preheat oven to 375°F and grease the baking dish.
2. Cut off tomatoes top, scoop out flesh, and chop.
3. Salt the inside and let them drain. Sauté onion in

olive oil until soft.

4. Add garlic, cook for 30 seconds. Add tomato flesh, salt, and cook until liquid evaporates.
5. Mix filling: Stir in tuna, olives, parsley, lemon juice, and pepper.
6. Fill tomatoes with mixture, top with lids if saved. Bake until tender.
7. Serve warm, room temp, or cold.

Mediterranean Fish Fillet

DAIRY FREE, GLUTEN FREE
PREP TIME: 10 MIN **COOK TIME:** 15 MIN **SERVINGS:** 6
Calories: 469, Carbs: 62g, Protein: 53g, Fat: 4g, Fiber: 2g, Sodium: 147mg

- 2 tsp ground coriander
- 2 tsp sumac
- 1½ tsp ground cumin
- 1 tsp dry dill weed
- 1 tsp turmeric
- 1 onion, chopped
- 8 garlic cloves, chopped
- 2 jalapeno peppers
- 5 ripe tomatoes, chopped
- 3 tbsp tomato paste
- 1 lime juice
- ½ cup water
- 2 lb cod fillet
- ½ cup chopped fresh parsley, to garnish
- 1 tbsp chopped fresh mint, to garnish

1. Mix coriander, sumac, cumin, dill, and turmeric.
2. Heat 2 tbsp oil in a skillet. Sauté onions for 2 minutes, then add garlic and jalapeño.
3. Cook until golden. Add tomatoes, half the spice mix, tomato paste, lime juice, water, salt, and pepper. Simmer for 10 minutes.
4. Season fish with salt, pepper, and remaining spice mix.
5. Add fish to the sauce. Cover and cook until flaky.
6. Garnish with parsley and mint. Serve with rice or bread.

Grilled Cod, Gyro-Style

GLUTEN FREE, DAIRY FREE
PREP TIME: 05 MIN **COOK TIME:** 20 MIN **SERVINGS:** 6
Calories: 327, Carbs: 11g, Protein: 33g, Fat: 17g, Fiber: 6g, Sodium: 187mg

Spice Rub:
- 1½ tsp dried oregano
- 1 tsp ground coriander
- 1 tsp ground cumin
- ½ tsp garlic powder
- ½ tsp sumac

For Fish:
- Olive oil
- 1.5 lb cod fillet
- Salt and pepper, to taste

Lemon Basil Sauce:
- ⅓ cup olive oil
- 1 juiced lemon
- 2 garlic cloves, minced
- 10 basil leaves, thinly chopped
- Salt and pepper, to taste

1. Combine spices for the spice rub.
2. Pat fish fillets dry, season with salt and pepper, and rub the spice mix all over. Set it aside.
3. Mix olive oil, lemon juice, garlic cloves, basil leaves, salt and pepper for the lemon basil sauce.
4. Set it aside. Prepare pita, Tzatziki sauce, and Mediterranean salad if serving.
5. Heat olive oil in a skillet over medium-high heat.
6. Cook fish fillets on each side until golden and crispy. Serve with a drizzle of lemon juice and lemon basil sauce.

Easy Mediterranean Sautéed Scallops

GLUTEN FREE, DAIRY FREE
PREP TIME: 10 MIN   COOK TIME: 13 MIN   SERVINGS: 4
Calories: 234 Carbs: 11g, Protein: 16g, Fat: 15g, Fiber: 2g, Sodium: 432mg

- 3 tbsp olive oil
- 1 shallot, sliced
- ½ red bell pepper, cut into thin strips
- 1 green bell pepper, cut into thin strips
- 5 garlic cloves, minced
- 10 oz grape tomato, halved
- 2 tbsp capers
- Black pepper, to taste
- ½ tsp oregano
- 1 tsp ground cumin
- ½ tsp paprika
- 2 tbsp olive oil
- 1 lb sea scallops
- Lemon to taste
- Fresh parsley for garnish

1. Heat 2-3 tbsp olive oil in a skillet. Sauté shallots and bell peppers.
2. Add garlic, tomatoes, capers, salt, pepper, oregano, cumin, and paprika.
3. Cook on low heat. In another skillet, heat 2 tbsp olive oil and sear scallops.
4. Add scallops to the vegetables, squeeze lemon juice over top, garnish with parsley, and serve.

Turkish-Style Marinated Salmon

DAIRY FREE, GLUTEN FREE
PREP TIME: 10 MIN   COOK TIME: 20 MIN   SERVINGS: 4
Calories: 386, Carbs: 3g, Protein: 34g, Fat: 27g, Fiber: 13g, Sodium: 382mg

- 2 tbsp olive oil
- 2 tbsp red pepper paste
- 2 tsp oregano
- 1 tsp smoked paprika
- 1 tbsp Aleppo pepper
- 1 tsp ground cumin
- 1 lemon juiced
- 4 garlic cloves
- Salt and pepper, to taste
- 2 lb salmon fillet
- Fresh herbs, for garnish

1. Marinate salmon with olive oil, spices, lemon juice, and garlic.
2. Refrigerate for 6 hours or overnight. Preheat oven to 375°F and line a sheet pan with foil.
3. Bake salmon, covered with foil. Broil to brown the top.
4. Serve garnished with fresh herbs.

Greek Salmon

GLUTEN FREE, DAIRY FREE
PREP TIME: 10 MIN   COOK TIME: 10 MIN   SERVINGS: 4
Calories: 182, Carbs: 5g, Protein: 24g, Fat: 8g, Fiber: 2g, Sodium: 622mg

- 2 tbsp olive oil
- 1 lemon, juiced
- 2 garlic cloves, minced
- 2 tsp Greek oregano
- 3 tbsp fresh dill, chopped
- 1 lb salmon fillet
- Salt, to taste
- Black pepper, to taste
- 2 green onions, chopped
- 1 cup cherry tomatoes

1. Preheat oven to 400°F and oil a baking dish. Mix lemon juice, zest, garlic, oregano, dill, and olive oil.
2. Season salmon with salt and pepper, place in dish, and top with green onions, tomatoes, and sauce.
3. Bake until flaky. Garnish with lemon zest and dill. Serve.

Persian Stuffed Fish

DAIRY FREE, GLUTEN FREE
PREP TIME: 05 MIN   COOK TIME: 25 MIN   SERVINGS: 4
Calories: 243, Carbs: 12g, Protein: 2g, Fat: 22g, Fiber: 3g, Sodium: 496mg

- 4 whole sea breams
- Salt a pinch
- Black pepper, a pinch
- ¼ cup walnuts
- 4 garlic cloves, crushed
- ½ cup fresh cilantro
- ½ cup parsley leaves
- 10 fresh mint leaves
- ⅔ cup green olives
- 2 tbsp pomegranate molasses
- ¼ cup olive oil
- 2 tbsp pomegranate seeds

1. Preheat oven to 400°F.
2. Line a baking sheet with foil. Score fish, season with salt and pepper, and place on the baking sheet.
3. Grind walnuts in a food processor. Add garlic, cilantro, parsley, and mint to walnuts, pulse until chopped.
4. Add olives, pomegranate molasses, and ¼ cup olive oil, pulse into a paste. Fill fish cavities with the walnut mixture.
5. Secure fish with butcher's twine. Drizzle with 2 tbsp olive oil.
6. Roast until crispy and cooked through. Remove twine, garnish with parsley and pomegranate seeds.

CHAPTER 10
POULTRY AND MEAT

From tender chicken to savory lamb, this chapter highlights the Mediterranean's love for flavorful, hearty meats. Infused with fresh herbs and spices, these dishes bring out the rich, comforting tastes of the region in every bite.

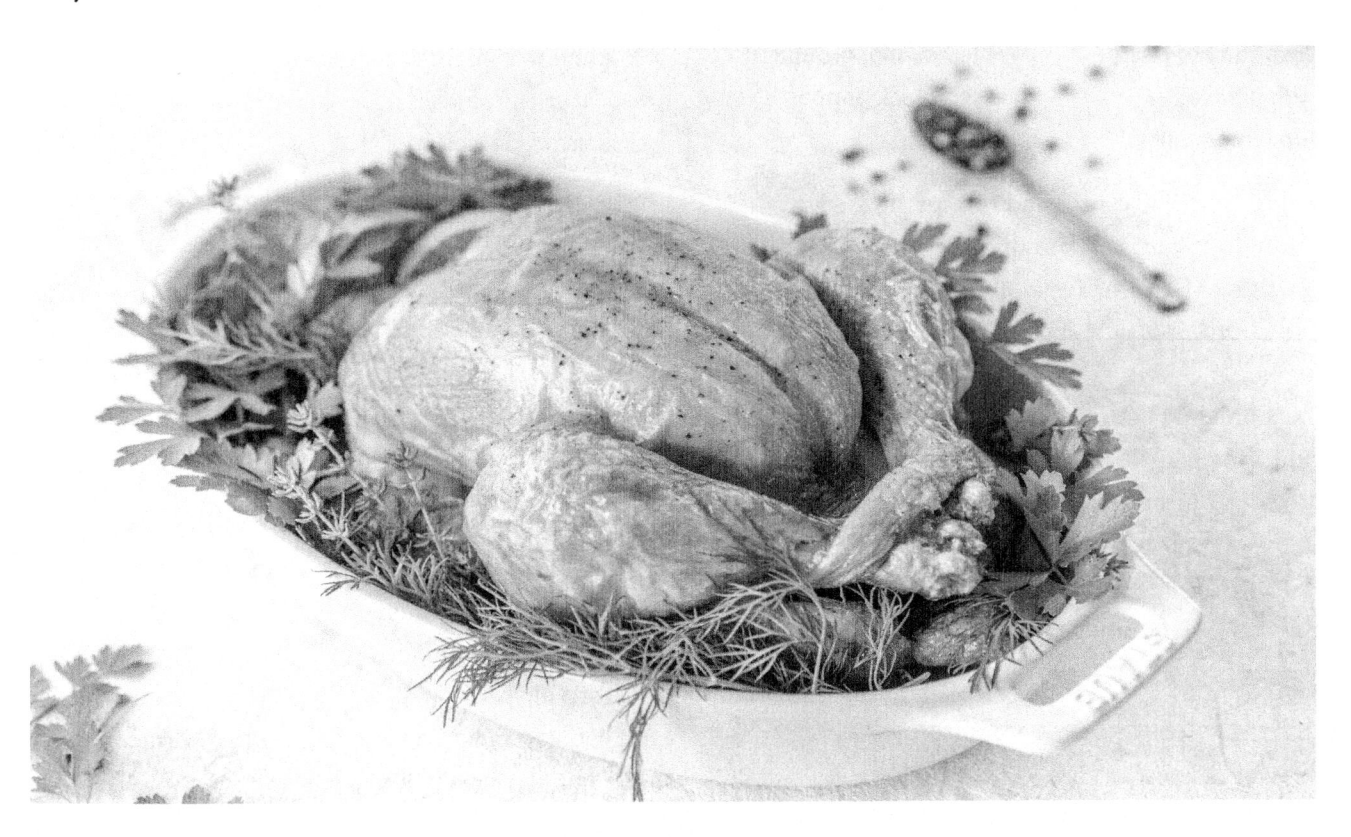

TIPS

- Boost your chicken or lamb with olive oil, garlic, lemon, and herbs. Let it sit for 30 minutes—or overnight—for maximum flavor!

- Fresh oregano, rosemary, thyme, and basil are your best friends! Add them to marinades or sprinkle on top for a burst of flavor.

- Olive oil is not just for cooking—drizzle over grilled meats or use in marinades to bring that rich, Mediterranean goodness to life.

Baked Chicken Thighs

GLUTEN FREE, DAIRY FREE
PREP TIME: 10 MIN **COOK TIME:** 25 MIN **SERVINGS:** 5
Calories: 313, Carbs: 9g, Protein: 20g, Fat: 29g, Fiber: 2g, Sodium: 337mg

- 8 bones in, chicken thighs
- Salt, to taste
- 1 vine ripe tomato, sliced
- ¼ cup water
- 5 tbsp tomato paste
- ⅓ cup olive oil
- 1 cup lemon, juiced
- 4 garlic cloves, chopped
- 3 onions, thinly sliced
- 1 tsp oregano, dried
- 1 tsp paprika, smoked
- 1 tsp cumin, grounded
- 1 tsp black pepper

1. Set racks to the center and top, preheat to 425°F.
2. Sprinkle salt on chicken thighs, including under the skin. Mix tomato paste, olive oil, lemon juice, garlic, oregano, smoked paprika, cumin, and pepper.
3. Coat chicken with rub, under and on top of the skin. Brush a 9x13" dish with olive oil.
4. Layer in onions, place chicken, add tomatoes, and pour water around edges.
5. Bake it. Broil for 1-3 minutes to brown.
6. Rest for 5-10 minutes, garnish with parsley, and serve.

Roast Turkey Breast

DAIRY FREE, GLUTEN FREE
PREP TIME: 10 MIN **COOK TIME:** 20 MIN **SERVINGS:** 5
Calories: 255, Carbs: 8g, Protein: 31g, Fat: 4g, Fiber: 2g, Sodium: 397mg

- 2 ½ lb bone-in turkey breast, half
- Salt, to taste
- 1 lb red grapes, stemmed
- ½ cup olive oil
- 1 tsp allspice
- 1 tsp paprika
- 1 tsp black pepper
- ½ tsp nutmeg
- 14 garlic cloves, minced
- Large handful parsley, chopped
- 8 small shallots, halved
- 7 celery stalks

1. Pat turkey dry, season with kosher salt, including under the skin. Let sit at room temperature.
2. Preheat oven to 450°F.
3. Take a pan and toss grapes with olive oil and salt, roast them. Set it aside.
4. Mix spices (allspice, paprika, black pepper, nutmeg). Rub on turkey, including under the skin. Coat with garlic, parsley, and olive oil mixture.
5. In the same pan in which you roasted grapes, add shallots and celery, season with salt and olive oil. Place turkey on top, skin side up.
6. Reduce oven to 350°F. Roast turkey then add grapes. Continue roasting until turkey reaches 155°F.
7. Cover turkey loosely with foil, let it rest until it reaches 165°F.
8. Carve turkey and slice. Serve with roasted grapes and vegetables.

Baked Tomato Chicken Thighs with Couscous

DAIRY FREE
PREP TIME: 05 MIN **COOK TIME:** 30 MIN **SERVINGS:** 6
Calories: 627, Carbs: 58g, Protein: 33g, Fat: 30g, Fiber: 6g, Sodium: 756mg

- 2 bell peppers, chopped
- 1 red onion, chopped
- 1 celery stalk, chopped
- 4 garlic cloves, minced
- 2 tbsp olive oil
- Salt and pepper, to taste
- 6 bone-in chicken thighs
- 1 tsp baharat spice
- 1 tsp turmeric
- 2 cups pearl couscous
- 2 cups vegetable broth
- 1 lemon, juiced and zest
- 1 bunch tarragon, chopped

1. Preheat oven to 400°F and position a rack in the center.
2. In a baking dish, toss bell peppers, onion, celery, garlic, olive oil, salt, and pepper.
3. Pat chicken thighs dry, season with salt, pepper, baharat, and turmeric. Rub spices in, then place chicken on top of vegetables, skin side down. Roast in the oven.
4. Remove chicken, stir in couscous, broth, lemon zest, lemon juice, and most of the tarragon (save some for garnish).
5. Place chicken skin side up on couscous mixture. Roast until chicken skin is crispy and couscous absorbs liquid.
6. Garnish with reserved tarragon and serve.

Greek Meatballs and Potatoes

DAIRY FREE
PREP TIME: 05 MIN **COOK TIME:** 25 MIN **SERVINGS:** 4
Calories: 332, Carbs: 27g, Protein: 27g, Fat: 12g,
Fiber: 4g, Sodium: 423mg

- 1 slice sandwich bread
- 1½ lb beef, grounded
- 1 yellow onion, chopped
- 2 garlic cloves, chopped
- 1 egg
- ¼ cup parsley, chopped
- 1 tsp oregano, dried
- 1 tsp coriander, grounded
- ½ tsp nutmeg
- Salt and pepper, to taste
- 4 Yukon gold potatoes, small chunks
- 1 red onion, chunks
- 1 batch ladolemono sauce

1. Set the oven to 375°F.
2. Soak bread with water, squeeze out excess liquid, and crumble it into a bowl.
3. Add beef, onion, garlic, egg, herbs, spices, salt, and pepper to bread. Combine.
4. Place potatoes and onions in a 9x13 pan.
5. Form the meatballs with the beef mix and place on top. Pour Ladolemono over.
6. Cover and bake. Uncover and bake.
7. Garnish with fresh herbs.

Sheet Pan Za'atar Chicken with Veggies

GLUTEN FREE, DAIRY FREE
PREP TIME: 10 MIN **COOK TIME:** 20 MIN **SERVINGS:** 4
Calories: 465, Carbs: 29g, Protein: 28g, Fat: 27g,
Fiber: 6g, Sodium: 654mg

- 2 tbsp za'atar
- 2 tsp sumac
- 1 tsp sweet paprika
- 6 garlic cloves, minced
- 2 lemons, juiced
- ½ cups olive oil
- Salt and pepper, to taste
- 5 Yukon gold potatoes, cut into large pieces
- 2 onions, halved and sliced into half moons
- 8 bone in, skin on chicken thighs

1. Preheat the oven to 425°F.
2. Mix za'atar, sumac, paprika, garlic, lemon juice, and olive oil.
3. Toss potatoes, and onions with salt, pepper, and 3-4 tbsp of the sauce. Spread on a sheet pan.
4. Rub chicken with salt, pepper, and remaining sauce under the skin.
5. Place chicken on veggies, drizzle with sauce. Cover with foil, bake.
6. Uncover, bake until crispy. Toss with olive oil, bake for 5 minutes.
7. Rest chicken for 5-10 minutes, garnish, and serve.

Pastilla (Skillet Chicken Pie)

DAIRY FREE
PREP TIME: 10 MIN **COOK TIME:** 20 MIN **SERVINGS:** 4
Calories: 382, Carbs: 36g, Protein: 28g, Fat: 15g,
Fiber: 3g, Sodium: 143mg

- 2 lb boneless chicken thighs
- Salt and pepper, to taste
- Olive oil
- 1 large onion, chopped
- 2 garlic cloves, minced
- 6 medjool dates, chopped
- ⅓ cup sliced almonds
- ½ cup parsley
- 3 eggs
- 10 sheets phyllo dough

Spice Mixture:
- 2 tsp Ras El Hanout
- 1 tsp cinnamon
- ½ tsp ground ginger
- ½ tsp red pepper flakes
- ¼ tsp turmeric

1. Season the chicken with salt and pepper. Sear in 2 tbsp olive oil for 5 minutes per side. Remove and set aside.
2. In the same pan, sauté onions and garlic with a pinch of salt until softened.
3. Add ¾ cup water and spices, bring to a boil. Return chicken to pan and cook until fully cooked and liquid reduces by half.
4. Remove chicken, shred it using forks, and return it to the pan.
5. Stir in beaten eggs, then add dates, almonds, and parsley. Remove from heat.
6. Preheat oven to 375°F and grease a 10-inch pie dish or skillet.
7. Brush and layer 8 sheets of phyllo dough (folded in half), overlapping in the pan.
8. Spread the chicken mixture on the phyllo, top with 2 more sheets of phyllo, and fold over edges.
9. Brush with olive oil and bake until phyllo is golden and crisp.

Roast Chicken with Citrus and Honey

GLUTEN FREE, DAIRY FREE

PREP TIME: 10 MIN **COOK TIME:** 20 MIN **SERVINGS:** 4

Calories: 616, Carbs: 45g, Protein: 28g, Fat: 38g,
Fiber: 5g, Sodium: 264mg

- 2 clementines
- 1 orange
- 1 lemon
- 2 garlic cloves, minced
- ½ cup olive oil
- ¼ cup honey
- 1 tbsp oregano
- 1 tsp thyme
- Salt and pepper, to taste
- 5 potatoes, sliced into wedges
- 2.5 lb whole chicken

1. Preheat oven to 400°F and line a baking sheet with parchment paper.
2. Juice clementines, orange, and lemon into a bowl. Add garlic, olive oil, honey, oregano, thyme, salt, and pepper. Whisk to combine.
3. Taste and add more salt or pepper if needed. Set aside.
4. Spread potato wedges on the baking sheet, season with salt and pepper, and set aside.
5. Remove the backbone with kitchen scissors, then flatten the chicken. Place it on top of the potatoes.
6. Pour marinade under the skin and over the chicken. Tuck peels of the fruits around the potatoes.
7. Roast, baste with pan juices, then cook until the internal temperature reaches 165°F.
8. Rest the chicken, carve, and serve with pan juices.

Italian Steak with Arugula and Parmesan

GLUTEN FREE, DAIRY FREE

PREP TIME: 10 MIN **COOK TIME:** 08 MIN **SERVINGS:** 4

Calories: 429, Carbs: 2g, Protein: 57g, Fat: 21g, Fiber: 1g, Sodium: 753mg

- 2 top sirloin steaks
- 2 tbsp olive oil
- 2 tsp salt, divided
- 3 oz arugula
- 2 tsp olive oil
- 2 tsp lemon, juiced
- 2 oz parmesan cheese (optional)

1. Preheat the grill to 500°F. Let the steaks sit at room temperature for 30 minutes.
2. Season steaks with olive oil and sea salt.
3. Grill for 3-4 minutes per side until internal temp reaches 140°F (medium rare).
4. Rest steaks, covered, for 5-10 minutes.
5. Toss arugula with olive oil, lemon juice, and salt.
6. Slice steaks, place on salad, top with parmesan.

Sun-Dried Tomato Chicken

GLUTEN FREE

PREP TIME: 10 MIN **COOK TIME:** 20 MIN **SERVINGS:** 4

Calories: 311, Carbs: 22g, Protein: 30g, Fat: 12g, Fiber: 3g, Sodium: 221mg

- 1 ½ lb chicken breasts
- 3 oz sun dried tomatoes, chopped
- 1 yellow onion, chopped
- 4 garlic cloves, minced
- Salt, to taste
- ⅓ cup white wine
- 1 ¾ cup whole milk
- 1 ½ tbsp cornstarch

1. Slice chicken breasts into cutlets, season with seasoning and salt.
2. Heat oil in a skillet, cook chicken for 4-6 minutes per side until 165°F. Set aside.
3. In the same skillet, sauté sun-dried tomatoes, onions, garlic, and salt.
4. Add wine, scrape browned bits. Stir in milk and cornstarch slurry, simmer until thick.
5. Add sliced chicken Plate chicken and sauce.

Pan Seared Lamb Chops

GLUTEN FREE, DAIRY FREE

PREP TIME: 10 MIN **COOK TIME:** 15 MIN **SERVINGS:** 4

Calories: 506, Carbs: 3g, Protein: 52g, Fat: 30g,
Fiber: 1g, Sodium: 282mg

- 8 lamb rib chops, trimmed
- 1 ¼ tsp kosher salt
- ½ tsp oregano, dried
- ¼ tsp black pepper
- Olive oil
- 3 garlic cloves, smashed
- 2 sprig thyme
- 2 sprig rosemary
- 1 lemon, zested

1. Rub chops with salt, oregano, and pepper. Heat oil, garlic, thyme, and rosemary in a hot skillet.

2. Cook chops 2-3 minutes per side, until 135°F internal temp.
3. Cover with foil, let rest for 5 minutes. Bake for 5 minutes.
4. Drizzle lamb with pan juices, garnish with garlic/herbs.
5. Sprinkle lamb chops with lemon zest. Serve with flatbread and yogurt sauce on the side.

Chicken Saltimbocca

GLUTEN FREE
PREP TIME: 10 MIN **COOK TIME:** 08 MIN **SERVINGS:** 4
Calories: 360, Carbs: 7g, Protein: 38g, Fat: 19g, Fiber: 0.2g, Sodium: 673mg

- 1 ½ lb chicken
- Salt and pepper, to taste
- ¼ cup gluten free flour
- 4 prosciutto slices
- 4 sage leaves, large
- ¼ cup white wine
- 2 tbsp butter

1. Slice and pound chicken breasts to ¼-inch thick. Season with salt and pepper.
2. Dredge in flour, top with prosciutto and sage, secure with a toothpick.
3. Heat oil in pan, cook cutlets 3 minutes per side until golden and cooked through. Put aside.
4. Add wine to pan, reduce by half, stir in butter, season with salt and pepper.
5. Return chicken to pan, remove toothpicks, and plate with sauce.

Stifado (Greek Beef Stew)

GLUTEN FREE, DAIRY FREE
PREP TIME: 10 MIN **COOK TIME:** 25 MIN **SERVINGS:** 4
Calories: 475, Carbs: 17g, Protein: 32g, Fat: 27g, Fiber: 4g, Sodium: 534mg

- 2 lb chuck roast
- ¾ tsp salt
- ½ tsp pepper
- ¼ cup olive oil
- 1 ½ lb whole pearl onions
- 5 garlic cloves, chopped
- 1 tbsp tomato paste
- 2 bay leaves
- 1 cinnamon stick
- ¼ tsp ground garlic clove
- 4 allspice berries
- ¼ cup cognac
- 1 can diced tomatoes

1. Pat beef dry, season with salt and pepper. Heat olive oil in a Dutch oven over high heat. Brown beef in batches until all pieces are seared. Transfer browned beef to a bowl and set aside.
2. Lower heat to medium, add pearl. Cook, stirring occasionally, until softened. Add garlic and cook for another minute.
3. Stir in tomato paste, bay leaves, cinnamon, ground clove, and allspice berries. Cook for 1 minute until fragrant.
4. Add browned beef and any juices back into the pot, stirring to coat with the spices and tomato paste.
5. Pour in cognac, scraping up any brown bits stuck to the bottom of the pot. Let it simmer.
6. Add canned tomatoes and enough warm water to cover the beef. Bring to a simmer, cover the pot, and cook on low until beef is tender. Stir halfway through and check liquid level, adding more water if needed.
7. Once beef is tender, taste and adjust seasoning. Remove bay leaves, cinnamon stick, and allspice berries. Let it rest and serve.

Greek Chicken Marinade

GLUTEN FREE, DAIRY FREE
PREP TIME: 05 MIN **COOK TIME:** 15 MIN **SERVINGS:** 4
Calories: 247, Carbs: 3g, Protein: 25g, Fat: 15g, Fiber: 1g, Sodium: 534mg

- 4 garlic cloves, minced
- 2 tsp dried oregano
- 1 tsp paprika
- 1 tsp thyme leaves
- 2 tbsp flat leaf parsley
- ⅓ cup olive oil
- 1 lemon, juiced and zested
- Salt and pepper, to taste
- 1 ½ to 2 lb chicken

1. Mix garlic, oregano, paprika, thyme, parsley, olive oil, lemon zest, juice, salt, and pepper.
2. Coat chicken, refrigerate. Preheat the oven to 400°F.
3. Slice chicken breasts into cutlets for even cooking.
4. Place chicken in a 9x13 dish, pour marinade over, cover with foil, and bake for 10 minutes.
5. Remove foil, bake until chicken reaches 160°F, about 10-15 minutes more.
6. Let the chicken rest for a while before serving.

Greek Meatloaf Wrapped in Grape Leaves

GLUTEN FREE, DAIRY FREE

PREP TIME: 10 MIN **COOK TIME:** 20 MIN **SERVINGS:** 5

Calories: 195, Carbs: 12g, Protein: 18g, Fat: 8g, Fiber: 3g, Sodium: 545mg

- 2 oz grape leaves
- 2 tbsp olive oil
- 1 onion, chopped
- 1 red bell pepper, chopped
- 2 garlic cloves, minced
- 1 lb lean beef
- 1 egg
- 2 tbsp tomato paste
- ½ cup mint leaves, chopped
- 1 tsp oregano, dried
- Salt and pepper, to taste
- 1 lemon

1. Preheat oven to 350°F. Coat a baking dish with olive oil.
2. Cook grape leaves for 3-5 minutes, then set aside. Sauté onion, bell pepper, and garlic in olive oil for 5-7 minutes.
3. Combine cooked veggies, ground beef, egg, tomato paste, mint, oregano, olive oil, salt, and pepper.
4. Shape mixture into a loaf, about 5 x 5 inches. Place grape leaves in the dish, put the meatloaf on top, and wrap with leaves.
5. Drizzle with olive oil, cover with foil, and bake for 20 mins. Squeeze lemon over meatloaf and let it rest.
6. Slice, garnish with parsley and tomatoes, and serve with lemon wedges.

Chicken in Tomato Sauce

GLUTEN FREE

PREP TIME: 10 MIN **COOK TIME:** 20 MIN **SERVINGS:** 4

Calories: 228, Carbs: 2g, Protein: 25g, Fat: 14g, Fiber: 0.5g, Sodium: 634mg

- 1 lb chicken breasts
- Salt, to taste
- Pepper, to taste
- 3 tbsp olive oil
- 1 garlic clove, minced
- 1 can whole tomatoes
- 1 tbsp capers
- Red pepper flakes, a pinch
- ½ tsp salt
- 2 tsp Italian seasoning
- 8 oz low moisture mozzarella

1. Slice and pound chicken to ¼-inch thick. Season with salt and pepper.
2. Heat 1 tbsp olive oil, cook garlic for 2-3 mins. Remove. Cook chicken cutlets 2 mins per side, set aside.
3. Add 2 tbsp olive oil, tomatoes, capers, red pepper flakes, and seasoning. Simmer for 5-8 mins.
4. Add chicken to pan, top with mozzarella, cover, cook 3-5 mins.
5. Plate chicken, spoon sauce over.

Garlic Dijon Chicken

GLUTEN FREE, DAIRY FREE

PREP TIME: 05 MIN **COOK TIME:** 25 MIN **SERVINGS:** 6

Calories: 198, Carbs: 4g, Protein: 16g, Fat: 12g, Fiber: 1g, Sodium: 156mg

- ½ lb boneless chicken thighs
- Salt and pepper, to taste
- 1 onion, roughly chopped
- Fresh parsley, chopped

For Garlic Dijon Sauce:
- 3 tsp Dijon mustard
- 2 tsp honey
- ⅓ cup olive oil
- 6 garlic cloves, minced
- 1 tsp coriander
- ¾ tsp paprika
- ½ tsp black pepper
- ½ tsp cayenne pepper
- Salt, a pinch

1. Preheat oven to 425°F.
2. Season chicken with salt and pepper on both sides, then set aside.
3. Mix Dijon mustard, honey, olive oil, garlic, spices, and salt in a bowl.
4. Coat chicken in sauce, then transfer to an oiled skillet or baking sheet. Add onions and drizzle with remaining sauce.
5. Bake until chicken reaches 165°F.
6. Garnish with parsley and serve.

Kleftiko (Greek Lamb Cooked in Parchment)

GLUTEN FREE, DAIRY FREE

PREP TIME: 10 MIN **COOK TIME:** 20 MIN **SERVINGS:** 4

Calories: 328, Carbs: 28g, Protein: 32g, Fat: 10g, Fiber: 4g, Sodium: 621mg

- 1 lamb boneless leg
- 2 ½ tbsp dried oregano
- 1 tbsp thyme
- 1 tbsp parsley

- Salt and pepper, to taste
- 1 tbsp Dijon mustard
- 10 garlic cloves, chopped
- 1 lemon, juiced
- 1 tbsp red wine vinegar
- ½ cup white wine
- ¼ cup olive oil
- 5 large russet potatoes, cubes
- 2 tomatoes, chopped
- 1 onion, chopped
- ½ cup vegetable broth
- 4 oz feta cheese, cut into blocks (optional)
- Olives, for garnishing

1. Rub lamb with oregano, thyme, parsley, salt, pepper, mustard, and garlic.
2. Place the lamb into a large bowl and then add lemon juice, vinegar, and ¼ cup olive oil. Marinate for at least 30 minutes or overnight.
3. Heat the oven to 375°F. Line the pan with parchment paper.
4. Spread potatoes, tomatoes, and onions in the pan. Season and drizzle with olive oil.
5. Place lamb on top and pour broth around it.
6. Fold and crimp parchment over lamb and veggies. Add feta cheese is using. Cook until tender, adding more broth if needed.
7. Rest, then shred lamb.
8. Add olives over it and serve.

Moroccan Meatballs

GLUTEN FREE, DAIRY FREE
PREP TIME: 15 MIN **COOK TIME:** 15 MIN **SERVINGS:** 4
Calories: 260, Carbs: 15g, Protein: 32g, Fat: 8g, Fiber: 3g, Sodium: 645mg

- 1 ¼ lb ground beef
- 1 onion, chopped
- 2 garlic cloves, minced
- Fresh cilantro leaves, chopped
- 3 tsp Ras El Hanout
- ½ tsp ground ginger
- ½ tsp cayenne
- Salt and pepper, to taste
- Olive oil

1. Add meat, onion, garlic, cilantro, Ras El Hanout, ginger, cayenne, salt, and pepper.
2. Mix well. Roll mixture into 1-inch balls. Place on tray, cover, refrigerate for 30 minutes.
3. Heat the pan over medium heat. Add oil, cook meatballs in batches for 7 minutes until cooked and charred.
4. Plate meatballs with carrot salad and sides. Enjoy!

Sausage and Lentils with Fennel

GLUTEN FREE, DAIRY FREE
PREP TIME: 05 MIN **COOK TIME:** 25 MIN **SERVINGS:** 4
Calories: 327, Carbs: 40g, Protein: 23g, Fat: 9g, Fiber: 4g, Sodium: 386mg

- 1 cup green lentils
- 3 cup water
- 8 oz chicken sausage
- Olive oil
- 1 fennel bulb, thinly sliced
- 2 large clove garlic, grated
- 1 yellow onion, chopped
- ½ tsp fennel seeds
- ½ cup broth
- 2 tbsp red wine vinegar

1. Simmer lentils in 3 cups of water for 10 minutes, partially covered.
2. Brown sausage in olive oil, breaking it up.
3. Add fennel, garlic, onion, carrots, broth, and vinegar to the sausage.
4. Add lentils to the skillet. Let it simmer.
5. Adjust seasoning, drizzle with olive oil, and serve with bread.

Moussaka

GLUTEN FREE
PREP TIME: 10 MIN **COOK TIME:** 20 MIN **SERVINGS:** 4
Calories: 240, Carbs: 7g, Protein: 18g, Fat: 15g, Fiber: 2g, Sodium: 270mg

- 1 medium eggplant, sliced into rounds
- ½ lb (250g) ground beef
- 1 cup diced tomatoes (canned or fresh)
- ½ cup grated Parmesan cheese
- 1 tbsp olive oil

1. Preheat the oven to 375°F (190°C). Lightly brush the eggplant slices with olive oil and grill or pan-fry until tender and slightly browned. Set aside.
2. In a skillet, cook the ground beef over medium heat until browned. Drain excess fat, then stir in the diced tomatoes. Simmer for 5 minutes.
3. In a baking dish, layer half the eggplant slices, followed by the beef mixture, then another layer of eggplant. Top with grated Parmesan cheese.
4. Bake in the preheated oven for 10–12 minutes, or until the cheese is melted and bubbly.
5. Serve warm with a side salad or crusty bread if desired.

Joojeh Kabob

GLUTEN FREE, DAIRY FREE

PREP TIME: 15 MIN **COOK TIME:** 15 MIN **SERVINGS:** 5

Calories: 251, Carbs: 3g, Protein: 38g, Fat: 10g, Fiber: 1g, Sodium: 189mg

- 2 ¼ lb boneless chicken breasts
- 1 onion, sliced
- 1 garlic clove, minced
- 1 large lemon, juiced
- ⅓ cup yogurt
- 2 tbsp olive oil
- 1 tbsp tomato puree
- ½ tsp turmeric
- Salt and pepper, to taste
- Parsley, chopped

1. Grind ¼ tsp saffron, mix with 3 tbsp water, let sit for 10 minutes.
2. Make marinade: Mix onion, garlic, lemon juice, yogurt, olive oil, tomato puree, turmeric, and saffron water.
3. Add chicken in marinade, season with salt and pepper, mix, cover, refrigerate overnight.
4. Thread marinated chicken(chopped into chunks) onto soaked skewers.
5. Cook on medium-high until 165°F internal temp. Garnish with parsley.

Shish Kabob

GLUTEN FREE, DAIRY FREE

PREP TIME: 20 MIN **COOK TIME:** 10 MIN **SERVINGS:** 5

Calories: 237, Carbs: 9g, Protein: 32g, Fat: 10g, Fiber: 3g, Sodium: 589mg

- 2 ½ tsp garlic powder
- 1 ½ ground nutmeg
- 1 ½ tsp ground green cardamom
- 1 tsp allspice
- 1 tsp paprika
- Salt and pepper, to taste
- 3 lb tenderloin fillet
- 1 onion, chopped
- 2 bell peppers
- 2 lemons, juiced
- 1 cup olive oil
- 1 cup dry red wine

1. Mix garlic powder, nutmeg, cardamom, allspice, paprika, salt, and pepper. Coat meat with spice rub.
2. Combine onions, 2/3 of lemon juice, olive oil, wine, with marinated meat. Refrigerate for 30 mins overnight.
3. Soak skewers (if bamboo), cut onion and peppers. Heat the pan on high for 10 minutes.
4. Thread meat (chopped into chunks), onion, and peppers onto skewers.
5. Cook kabobs for 8-10 minutes, brushing with rest of the lemon juice. Let kabobs rest for 5 minutes. Enjoy!

Baked Boneless Chicken Thighs with Baharat

GLUTEN FREE, DAIRY FREE

PREP TIME: 05 MIN **COOK TIME:** 30 MIN **SERVINGS:** 5

Calories: 324, Carbs: 17g, Protein: 24g, Fat: 19g, Fiber: 3g, Sodium: 583mg

- 1 lb potatoes
- 1 lemon, juiced
- 3 shallots, halved
- 8 skinless chicken thighs
- 3 tbsp sesame seeds
- ½ cup olive oil
- 5 garlic cloves, minced
- 4 tbsp tomato paste
- 2 tsp baharat
- ½ tsp red pepper flakes

1. Preheat the oven to 425°F, center rack. Mix lime juice, olive oil, garlic, tomato paste, Baharat, and red pepper flakes.
2. Toss potatoes with ¼ cup marinade, salt. Place in an oiled pan with shallots. Bake potatoes.
3. Season chicken with salt, toss in marinade.
4. Let sit for 15 minutes. Toast sesame seeds in a hot skillet until golden. Set it aside.
5. Add chicken to the pan, bake, until cooked.
6. Top with sesame seeds and parsley. Serve!

Skillet Mushroom Chicken

GLUTEN FREE, DAIRY FREE

PREP TIME: 10 MIN **COOK TIME:** 10 MIN **SERVINGS:** 5

Calories: 256, Carbs: 5g, Protein: 32g, Fat: 13g, Fiber: 1g, Sodium: 632mg

- 1 ½ lb boneless chicken breasts
- Salt and pepper, to taste
- 1 tsp oregano
- 1 tsp paprika
- 1 tsp coriander
- 2 tbsp olive oil
- 1 tbsp ghee
- 12 oz white button mushrooms
- ½ cup chicken broth
- 3 green onions, chopped
- 2 garlic cloves, minced
- Salt and pepper, to taste

1. Preheat the oven to 200°F. Slice chicken into thin

cutlets, season with salt, pepper, oregano, paprika, and coriander.
2. Heat oil in a skillet. Cook chicken 3-4 minutes per side, transfer to an ovenproof dish, and keep warm in the oven.
3. In the same skillet, heat oil and ghee. Sauté mushrooms for 5 minutes.
4. Add broth, green onions, garlic, salt, and pepper. Boil.
5. Return chicken to skillet, spoon sauce over, and serve.

Greek Lamb Stew with Orzo

GLUTEN FREE, DAIRY FREE
PREP TIME: 10 MIN **COOK TIME:** 20 MIN **SERVINGS:** 5
Calories: 198, Carbs: 22g, Protein: 13g, Fat: 3g, Fiber: 1g, Sodium: 468mg

- 1 lb lamb
- Salt and pepper, to taste
- 3 tbsp olive oil
- 2 onions, chopped
- 4 garlic cloves, chopped
- 1 cup red wine
- 1 tsp dry oregano
- 1 tsp paprika
- ½ tsp ground cinnamon
- ½ tsp nutmeg
- 1 bay leaf
- 28 oz chopped San Marzano tomatoes
- 1 cup orzo pasta
- ½ cup parsley

1. Pat dry lamb, season with salt and pepper.
2. Heat olive oil in a pan. Brown lamb, set aside. In the same pan, cook onions and garlic with salt. Simmer.
3. Add lamb, wine, spices, and tomatoes. Let it simmer. Stir in orzo, cook.
4. Garnish with parsley and feta (optional).

Italian Meatballs in Tomato Sauce

GLUTEN FREE
PREP TIME: 10 MIN **COOK TIME:** 25 MIN **SERVINGS:** 4
Calories: 105, Carbs: 9g, Protein: 6g, Fat: 5g, Fiber: 2g, Sodium: 286mg

- 1 lb beef
- 2 tbsp parsley leaves
- 1 garlic clove, minced
- 1 egg
- 2 tbsp parmesan cheese
- Salt, to taste
- ¼ cup tbsp olive oil
- ½ yellow onions, chopped
- 2 tbsp pecorino Romano cheese
- 2 tbsp dry white wine
- 5 cups tomato puree (passata)
- Pinch red pepper flakes
- Handful basil leaves

1. Combine beef, parsley, garlic, egg, cheese, wine, and salt.
2. Shape into 12 balls and place on a parchment-lined plate.
3. Heat 2 tbsp oil, brown meatballs in batches (5 minutes each). Set it aside. Cook onions in 2 tbsp oil until soft (5 minutes).
4. Add passata, red pepper flakes, and 1 cup water from the passata container.
5. Return meatballs to sauce, let it simmer. Stir in basil, serve with parmesan.

Moroccan-Inspired Chicken Couscous

GLUTEN FREE, DAIRY FREE
PREP TIME: 15 MIN **COOK TIME:** 15 MIN **SERVINGS:** 4
Calories: 492, Carbs: 32g, Protein: 24g, Fat: 8g, Fiber: 4g, Sodium: 388mg

- ⅓ cup olive oil
- 1 tbsp red wine vinegar
- 3 tbsp tomato paste
- 4 clove garlic, minced
- 2 tsp Ras el Hanout
- 1 tsp ground cinnamon
- ¾ tsp ground ginger
- 8 chicken thighs
- 1 red onion, halved cut into small pieces
- 1 cup couscous
- 1 cup water
- ½ tsp ground cinnamon
- 1 cup parsley

1. Preheat the oven to 425°F. Combine olive oil, vinegar, tomato paste, garlic, and spices in a bowl.
2. Pat chicken dry, season with salt and pepper, and coat with 3/4 of the rub.
3. Toss vegetables and onions with salt, pepper, and the remaining rub. Place chicken and veggies in a pan and bake until cooked through.
4. Toast couscous in olive oil. Add boiling water, cinnamon, and salt. Cover for 10 minutes.
5. Fluff couscous with parsley, then serve with chicken and veggies.
6. Optional: Add raisins.

Apricot Chicken

GLUTEN FREE, DAIRY FREE
PREP TIME: 05 MIN **COOK TIME:** 20 MIN **SERVINGS:** 5
Calories: 356, Carbs: 22g, Protein: 18g, Fat: 23g, Fiber: 3g, Sodium: 185mg

- ½ cup dried apricots
- ½ tsp saffron
- 4 chicken thighs (bone-in, skin-on)
- 3 tbsp olive oil
- Salt and pepper, to taste
- 2 tsp spice blend (turmeric, coriander, cumin, cinnamon)
- 1 onion, diced
- 4 garlic cloves, minced

1. Soak apricots in warm water. Bloom saffron in water.
2. Sear chicken in oil, season with salt, pepper, and half the spice blend. Set it aside.
3. Cook onion, garlic, and spices in the same pan. Add chopped apricots, and saffron water.
4. Simmer for 10 minutes. Preheat the oven to 400°F.
5. Place chicken in sauce and roast. Serve.

Chicken Tagine

GLUTEN FREE, DAIRY FREE
PREP TIME: 10 MIN **COOK TIME:** 20 MIN **SERVINGS:** 4
Calories: 210, Carbs: 5g, Protein: 23g, Fat: 11g, Fiber: 1g, Sodium: 350mg

- 2 chicken thighs (bone-in or boneless)
- 1 cup diced tomatoes (canned or fresh)
- ½ cup chicken broth
- ¼ cup green olives, pitted
- 1 tbsp olive oil
- 1 tsp ground cumin

1. Heat olive oil in a large skillet or tagine pot over medium heat. Add the chicken thighs and sear for 2–3 minutes per side until golden brown.
2. Remove the chicken and set it aside. In the same skillet, add diced tomatoes, chicken broth, and ground cumin. Stir well.
3. Return the chicken to the skillet and add the green olives. Cover and simmer over low heat for 15–18 minutes, or until the chicken is fully cooked and tender.
4. Serve warm, garnished with fresh herbs if desired.

Albondigas (Spanish Meatballs)

DAIRY FREE
PREP TIME: 10 MIN **COOK TIME:** 20 MIN **SERVINGS:** 4
Calories: 401, Carbs: 17g, Protein: 28g, Fat: 24g, Fiber: 3g, Sodium: 487mg

- 1 ½ lb ground beef
- 1 onion, chopped
- 2 garlic cloves, minced
- 1 egg
- ¼ parsley, chopped
- 1 tsp salt
- ¼ cup olive oil

For Sofrito:
- 1 onion, chopped
- 4 garlic cloves, minced
- 1 cup canned tomatoes, chopped
- ½ tsp salt
- ¼ cup parsley
- 1 tsp unsalted almonds
- 1 cup chicken broth

1. In a bowl, mix ground beef, chopped onion, minced garlic, egg, parsley, salt, and pepper. Mix gently.
2. Shape the mixture into meatballs
3. Sprinkle flour over the meatballs and roll to coat evenly.
4. Heat olive oil. Fry half the meatballs until browned on all sides. Remove and drain on paper towels. Repeat with the remaining meatballs.
5. To make sofrito, discard most oil from the pan, leaving 2 tbsp. Add chopped onion and sauté for 5 minutes. Add garlic, cook for 1 minute. Stir in tomato and salt, cook until liquid reduces.
6. Add chicken stock to the sofrito. Add meatballs, reduce heat, and simmer for 5-10 minutes, until the sauce thickens.
7. Serve with crusty bread or over rice.

Scan this QR code to download recipes with vibrant, full-color photos - '**A Reference Book of 70 Classic Mediterranean Recipes with Full Colored Pictures**'

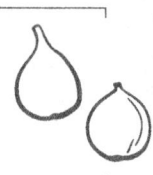

CHAPTER 11
EGGS

Eggs are a Mediterranean must-have, and it's easy to see why! From shakshuka to spanakopita, they're super versatile and full of flavor. In this chapter, we'll dive into how the Mediterranean uses eggs in everything from quick breakfasts to hearty dinners. Let's crack on and get cooking!

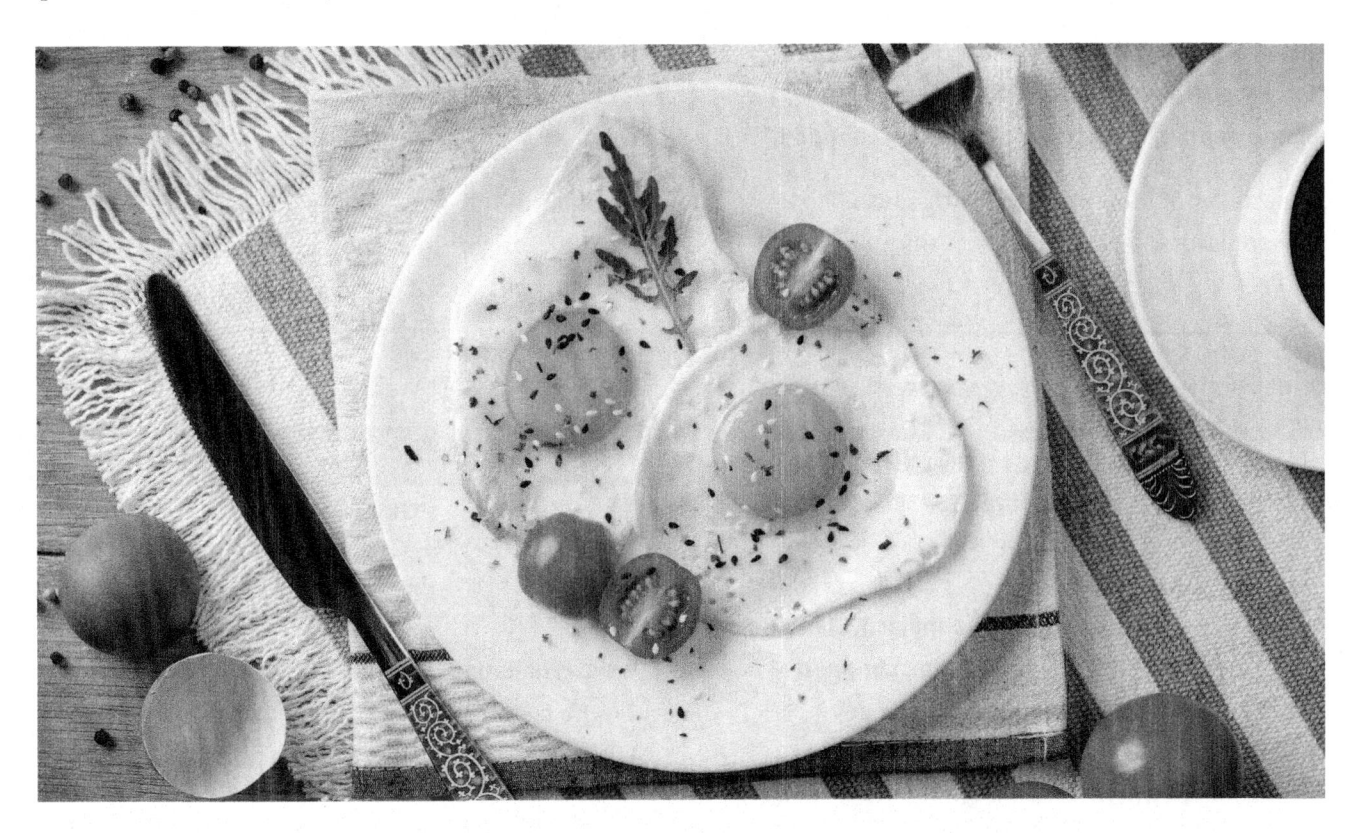

TIPS

- Instead of butter, cook eggs in olive oil for a richer, healthier Mediterranean twist.

- Always season your eggs with salt and pepper before cooking for even flavor throughout.

- From omelets to baked dishes like frittatas, eggs are the perfect way to add protein and flavor to any Mediterranean meal.

White Bean Shakshuka

VEGETARIAN

PREP TIME: 05 MIN **COOK TIME:** 25 MIN **SERVINGS:** 4

Calories: 115, Carbs: 12g, Fat: 5g, Protein: 8g, Fiber: 2g, Sodium: 221mg

- 1 onion, halved
- 2 garlic cloves, chopped
- 1 tsp ground coriander
- 1 tsp paprika
- ½ tsp cumin
- ½ tsp Aleppo pepper
- Salt and pepper, to taste
- 1 can (28 oz) diced tomatoes
- 1 can (15 oz) cannellini beans, drained
- 4 eggs
- ¼ cup parsley, chopped
- ¼ cup dill, chopped

1. Heat oil, cook onions, garlic with spices.
2. Add tomatoes, beans, boil, then simmer.
3. Make wells, crack eggs, cover, cook.
4. Drizzle with olive oil, add herbs, and serve.

Spanakopita Egg Muffins

VEGETARIAN, GLUTEN FREE

PREP TIME: 05 MIN **COOK TIME:** 25 MIN **SERVINGS:** 6

Calories: 139, Carbs: 4g, Fat: 8g, Protein: 12g, Fiber: 5g, Sodium: 146mg

- 12 eggs
- 1 ½ tsp oregano
- ¾ tsp black pepper
- ¾ tsp paprika
- ¼ tsp baking powder
- Salt, to taste
- 9 oz spinach, chopped
- ¾ onion, chopped
- 1 ¼ cup parsley
- ¼ cup mint leaves
- 4 garlic cloves, minced
- 6 oz feta cheese

1. Preheat oven to 350°F, grease muffin tin.
2. Whisk eggs, spices, baking powder, salt, spinach, onion, herbs, garlic, and feta.
3. Fill muffin cups 3/4 full, bake for 25-30 minutes.
4. Cool slightly, loosen with a knife, remove, and serve or store.

Italina Eggs in Purgatory

VEGETARIAN, GLUTEN FREE

PREP TIME: 10 MIN **COOK TIME:** 25 MIN **SERVINGS:** 4

Calories: 208, Carbs: 10g, Fat: 16g, Protein: 8g, Fiber: 2g, Sodium: 257mg

- 3 tbsp olive oil
- 1 onion, chopped
- 1 garlic clove, minced
- Pinch of red pepper flakes
- 2 tsp red pepper flakes
- 1 red bell pepper, chopped
- 28 oz tomatoes, chopped
- 4 eggs
- 5-8 basil leaves
- 3-4 tsp parmigiano

1. Cook onion, garlic, red pepper flakes, and bell pepper in oil.
2. Season. Stir in tomatoes, let it simmer.
3. Make wells, crack eggs, cover and cook. Garnish with basil and cheese.
4. Serve with bread.

Halloumi Cheese with Egg

GLUTEN FREE

PREP TIME: 05 MIN **COOK TIME:** 10 MIN **SERVINGS:** 2

Calories: 230, Carbs: 1g, Fat: 19g, Protein: 14g, Fiber: 0g, Sodium: 450mg

- 4 slices halloumi cheese
- 2 large eggs
- 1 tbsp olive oil
- ¼ tsp black pepper
- 1 tbsp fresh parsley, chopped

1. Heat olive oil in a non-stick pan over medium heat. Add halloumi slices and cook for 2 minutes on each side until golden brown.
2. Push the halloumi to the side of the pan and crack the eggs into the center. Sprinkle black pepper on top.
3. Cook until the egg whites are set but the yolks are still runny, about 3–4 minutes.
4. Serve the eggs and halloumi together, garnished with fresh parsley.

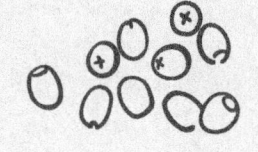

Dijon Deviled Eggs

VEGETARIAN, GLUTEN FREE
PREP TIME: 10 MIN **COOK TIME:** 15 MIN **SERVINGS:** 12
Calories: 35, Carbs: 1g, Fat: 2, Protein: 4g, Fiber: 1g, Sodium: 37mg

- 6 eggs
- ¼ yogurt
- 1 tsp Dijon mustard
- Salt, to taste
- ½ tsp garlic powder
- 2 tbsp chives, chopped
- Capers, for garnish

1. Boil eggs, turn off heat, cover, let sit for 10 minutes.
2. Drain, run under cold water. Peel and slice eggs in half. Scoop out yolks and mix it with yogurt, mustard, garlic powder, and salt.
3. Pipe or spoon filling into egg whites. Garnish with paprika, chives, and capers.
4. Serve or refrigerate.

Turkish Poached Eggs

VEGETARIAN, GLUTEN FREE
PREP TIME: 10 MIN **COOK TIME:** 10 MIN **SERVINGS:** 2
Calories: 343, Carbs: 7g, Fat: 6g, Protein: 18g, Fiber: 1g, Sodium: 142mg

- 1 cup yogurt
- 1-2 garlic cloves, minced
- Salt, to taste
- 2 eggs
- 3 tbsp olive oil
- 2 tsp white vinegar
- 2 tsp Aleppo pepper

1. Mix yogurt, garlic, and salt. Divide into two bowls.
2. Boil water with vinegar. Drain egg whites, add egg to vortex, cook 2-3 mins.
3. Repeat for the second egg. Heat olive oil and Aleppo pepper in a skillet.
4. Place eggs on yogurt, drizzle with oil. Enjoy with bread.

Eggs Fra Diavolo

VEGETARIAN, GLUTEN FREE
PREP TIME: 05 MIN **COOK TIME:** 15 MIN **SERVINGS:** 6
Calories: 102, Carbs: 6g, Fat: 8g, Protein: 6g, Fiber: 2g, Sodium: 200mg

- 6 eggs, hard boiled
- 1 onion, chopped
- 5 garlic cloves, minced
- 1 hot pepper, chopped
- Salt, to taste
- 5 oz roasted tomatoes, chopped
- ¼ cup tomato paste
- 2 tsp dried oregano
- 1-2 tsp red pepper flakes
- ½ cup parsley, chopped

1. Heat oil, cook eggs until crispy. Set aside.
2. Sauté onions, hot pepper, and garlic. Season with salt.
3. Add tomatoes, paste, water, seasonings. Let it simmer. Add eggs and cook.
4. Garnish with parsley, drizzle oil, and serve with bread.

Tuna Deviled Eggs

GLUTEN FREE
PREP TIME: 10 MIN **COOK TIME:** 15 MIN **SERVINGS:** 6
Calories: 228 Carbs: 1g Fat: 17g Protein: 16g Fiber: 1g Sodium: 387mg

- 6 eggs
- 7 oz tuna canned, drained
- 5 tbsp mayonnaise
- 12 green olives, chopped
- ¼ tsp black pepper
- ¼ tsp paprika
- Salt, to taste
- Parsley, for garnish

1. Boil eggs for 10-12 minutes, cool in cold water, peel, and half.
2. Mash mayo, tuna, olives, pepper, and paprika together. Add yolks to mixture, mix well.
3. Spoon filling into whites, sprinkle with paprika, salt, and parsley.
4. Refrigerate for 30 minutes.

Lebanese Potatoes and Eggs

GLUTEN FREE, VEGETARIAN
PREP TIME: 05 MIN **COOK TIME:** 15 MIN **SERVINGS:** 4
Calories: 265, Carbs: 19g, Fat: 18g, Protein: 7g, Fiber: 2g, Sodium: 344mg

- 2 potatoes, peeled
- 3 boiled eggs, peeled
- 1 tsp lemon juice
- 4 tbsp olive oil
- ½ tsp salt
- ½ tsp black pepper
- Parsley, for garnish

1. Boil potatoes for 8-10 minutes until tender. Mash potatoes and eggs.
2. Add lemon juice, olive oil, salt, and pepper.
3. Drizzle with olive oil and garnish with parsley.

Tunisian Brik au Thon

VEGETARIAN, DAIRY FREE

PREP TIME: 10 MIN **COOK TIME:** 20 MIN **SERVINGS:** 4

Calories: 335, Carbs: 33g, Fat: 16g, Protein: 17g, Fiber: 4g, Sodium: 952mg

- ½ lb potatoes, peeled
- 2 tbsp olive oil
- Salt and pepper, to taste
- 1 cup parsley, chopped
- 8 sheets filo dough
- 5 oz canned tuna
- ½ cup capers, rinsed
- 4 eggs
- 1 lemon

1. Boil potatoes with salt, then drain. Mash with olive oil, salt, pepper, and parsley. Let cool.
2. Place 2 sheets on a plate. Fold them in half and roll the sides toward the center to form a square shape.
3. Place ¼ mashed potato, crack an egg in the center, top with tuna and capers.
4. Moisten edges, fold into a triangle, and press to seal. Repeat for remaining ingredients.
5. Heat oil, fry Brik until golden and yolk is runny.
6. Drain Brik on paper towels, then serve with lemon, capers, and parsley.

Turkish Spinach and Eggs

VEGETARIAN, GLUTEN FREE

PREP TIME: 10 MIN **COOK TIME:** 20 MIN **SERVINGS:** 4

Calories: 168, Carbs: 9g, Fat: 12g, Protein: 9g, Fiber: 3g, Sodium: 127mg

- 2 tbsp olive oil
- 1 onion, diced
- 3 garlic cloves, crushed
- ½ tsp ground cumin
- ¼ tsp smoked paprika
- 2 tbsp Turkish sweet red pepper paste
- 2 tomatoes, chopped
- ⅓ cup water
- 10 oz spinach
- Salt and pepper, to taste
- 4 eggs
- ½ tsp Aleppo pepper

1. Heat oil, cook onions. Stir in cumin, paprika, and red pepper paste.
2. Add tomatoes, water, and spinach.
3. Cook for 7 mins, season. Make wells, crack eggs, cover, cook for 5-7 mins.
4. Garnish with Aleppo pepper and parsley.

Soft Scrambled Eggs with Chives

VEGETARIAN, GLUTEN FREE

PREP TIME: 02 MIN **COOK TIME:** 08 MIN **SERVINGS:** 2

Calories: 206, Carbs: 2g, Fat: 16g, Protein: 13g, Fiber: 1g, Sodium: 30mg

- 4 eggs
- Salt, to taste
- Olive oil, to taste
- 2-3 tsp yogurt
- 1 tsp chives, chopped

1. Whisk eggs with salt and olive oil.
2. Heat olive oil in a skillet for 30 seconds. Stir eggs in skillet until they begin to set.
3. Stir in yogurt, combine until set. Adjust seasoning.
4. Plate, garnish with chives. Serve.

Za'atar Olive Oil Fried Eggs

VEGETARIAN, GLUTEN FREE

PREP TIME: 01 MIN **COOK TIME:** 02 MIN **SERVINGS:** 1

Calories: 193, Carbs: 2g, Fat: 3g, Protein: 6g, Fiber: 1g, Sodium: 645mg

- 1 egg
- 1-2 tbsp olive oil
- ¼ tsp salt
- 2 tsp za'atar

1. Crack egg into a ramekin. Warm skillet, add oil, swirl to coat.
2. Slide in egg, season with salt and za'atar, cook 2-3 minutes, spoon oil over egg.
3. Serve with pita or crusty bread.

Oven Baked Eggs

VEGETARIAN, DAIRY FREE

PREP TIME: 05 MIN **COOK TIME:** 08 MIN **SERVINGS:** 2

Calories: 126, Carbs: 1g, Fat: 8g, Protein: 12g, Fiber: 3g, Sodium: 415mg

- 4 eggs
- Salt and pepper, to taste
- Olive oil, to taste
- Toppings, of your choice

1. Preheat oven to 375°F, middle rack.
2. Brush ramekins with olive oil.
3. Crack 1 egg per ramekin. Place on a sheet pan, bake 8 mins (2 extra for firmer yolks).
4. Season, add toppings, serve.

CHAPTER 12

BAKED GOODS - BREADS, FLATBREADS, PIZZAS, WRAPS

Welcome to the world of Mediterranean baked goods—from warm, crusty breads to flaky flatbreads, pizzas, and wraps! Whether you're dipping, wrapping, or topping, these baked treats are the heart of Mediterranean cuisine.

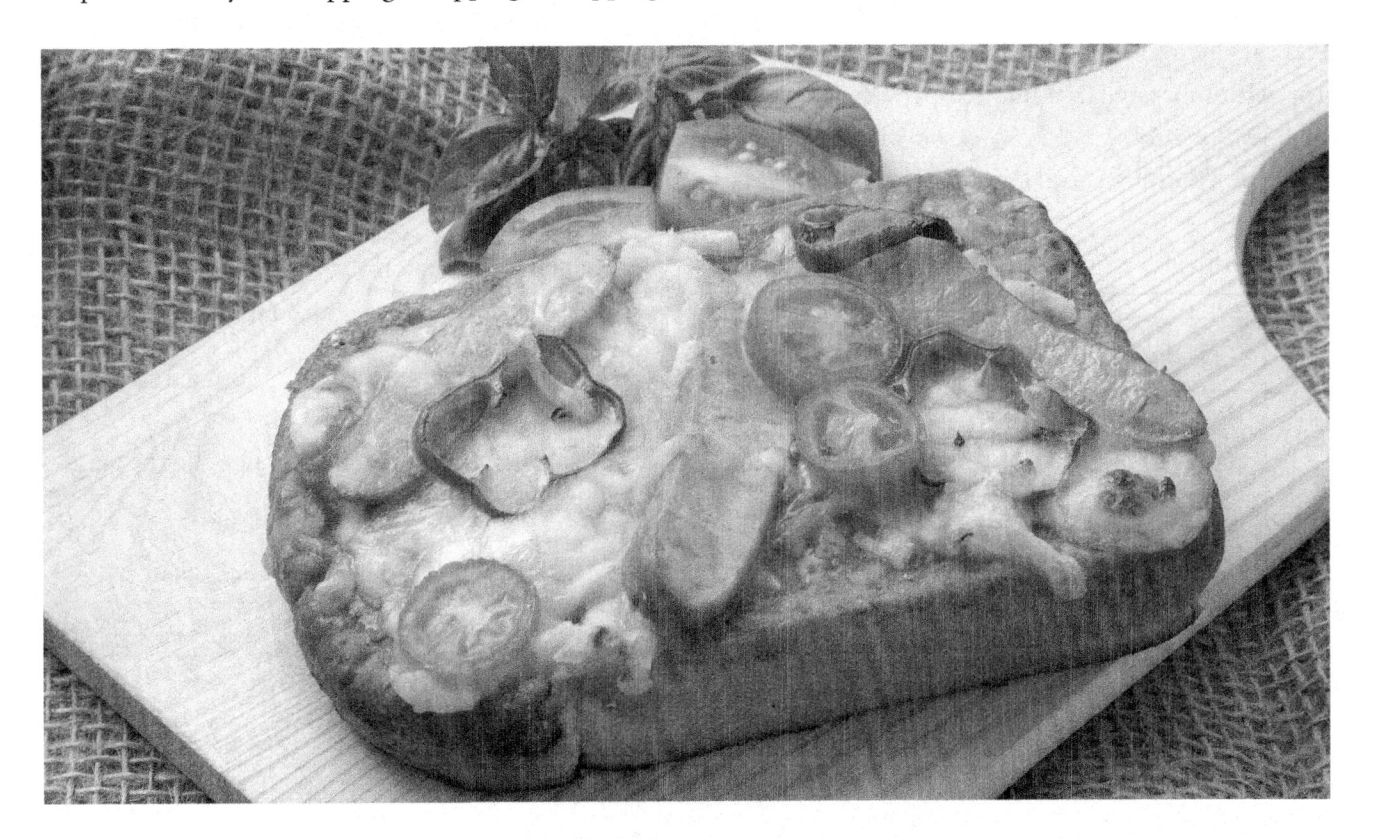

TIPS

- Try semolina or whole wheat for a denser, more Mediterranean-style bread, especially in flatbreads.

- Swap olive oil for butter in dough for a richer, moist, Mediterranean twist.

- For a sweet touch, mix in honey or dates to your dough, perfect for Mediterranean flatbreads.

Pita Breakfast Pizza

VEGETARIAN
PREP TIME: 05 MIN **COOK TIME:** 05 MIN
SERVINGS: 10
Calories: 84, Carbs: 7g, Fat: 5g, Protein: 6g, Fiber: 1g, Sodium: 119mg

- 1 pita bread
- Olive oil, to taste
- ½ cup mozzarella
- 1 tsp za'atar
- 1 shallot, chopped
- 1 Roma tomato, chopped
- 2 eggs, boiled
- Salt, to taste

1. Preheat the oven to 375°F. Brush pita with olive oil.
2. Top with mozzarella, za'atar, red pepper flakes, shallots, tomatoes, and egg. Season with salt.
3. Bake for 5 minutes until cheese melts and edges crisp.
4. Serve with extra za'atar and enjoy it hot.

Vegetarian Pizza

VEGETARIAN
PREP TIME: 10 MIN **COOK TIME:** 25 MIN **SERVINGS:** 8
Calories: 301, Carbs: 34g, Fat: 15g, Protein: 10g, Fiber: 3g, Sodium: 484mg

- 1 cup warm water
- 2 ¼ tsp dry yeast
- 1 tsp sugar
- 2 ¼ cups flour
- 1 tsp sea salt
- 3 tbsp olive oil
- 1 onion, chopped
- 4 garlic cloves, chopped
- 8 oz cremini mushrooms, chopped
- 1 red bell pepper, sliced
- 5 oz spinach leaves
- ⅓ cup feta cheese
- 1 tsp Aleppo pepper
- 1 egg, beaten
- 1 tbsp olive oil, to brush

1. Set the oven to 400°F. Line two baking sheets with parchment.
2. Mix warm water, yeast, and sugar. Let sit 5-8 minutes until frothy.
3. Combine flour, salt, olive oil, and yeast mixture. Stir into a sticky dough.
4. Knead on floured surface for 3-4 minutes until smooth.
5. Coat dough in olive oil, cover, and let rise for 1 hour.
6. Sauté onions, garlic, peppers, and mushrooms in olive oil. Add spinach, feta, and Aleppo pepper. Cool.
7. Divide dough into 2 balls. Roll each into 8x16-inch oval.
8. Spread filling on one dough, fold edges, and pinch ends. Repeat with second dough.
9. Brush edges with egg wash. Bake until golden.
10. Slice and enjoy!

Mediterranean Wrap

VEGETARIAN, DAIRY FREE
PREP TIME: 08 MIN **COOK TIME:** 00 MIN **SERVINGS:** 1
Calories: 210 Carbs: 12g Fat: 8g Protein: 7g Fiber: 3g Sodium: 210mg

- 1 cup cooked white beans
- ¼ tsp salt
- ¾ tsp granulated onion
- ⅛ tsp garlic powder
- 1 tbsp olive oil
- 1 ½ tsp lemon juice
- 10-inches wraps
- Toppings of your choice

1. Mash white beans with salt, onion, garlic powder, olive oil and lemon juice.
2. Spread the mix on wraps. Arrange the toppings of your choice.
3. Roll the wrap and close it.

Majorcan Vegetable Flatbread

VEGETARIAN
PREP TIME: 10 MIN **COOK TIME:** 20 MIN **SERVINGS:** 8
Calories: 317, Carbs: 27g, Fat: 21g, Protein: 5g, Fiber: 2g, Sodium: 315mg

- 2 cups flour
- ½ tsp bread yeast
- 1 egg
- 1 tbsp butter
- ½ cup olive oil
- 1 tsp salt
- ½ tsp sugar
- ½ warm water
- 1 green bell pepper, diced
- 2 tomatoes, diced
- 1 onion, diced
- 1 tsp parsley
- 1 tsp paprika
- 3 tbsp olive oil
- Parsley (optional)

1. Preheat the oven to 375°F.
2. In a bowl, combine flour, yeast, egg, butter, ½ cup olive oil, salt, and sugar.
3. Gradually add water and mix. Knead until smooth. Let's rest.
4. Dice pepper, tomatoes, onion. Mix with parsley,

paprika, salt, pepper, and 3 tbsp olive oil.
5. Roll out dough on a baking sheet, pressing from the center out.
6. Spread salad mix on dough. Bake at 375°F for 15 minutes. Increase to 400°F for 5 more minutes.
7. Top with parsley. Cut into and serve.

Palestinian Flatbread

VEGETARIAN

PREP TIME: 10 MIN **COOK TIME:** 20 MIN **SERVINGS:** 4
Calories: 536, Carbs: 98g, Fat: 10g, Protein: 17g, Fiber: 8g, Sodium: 878mg

- **1 ⅓ cup warm water**
- **2 ½ instant yeast**
- **1 ½ tsp sugar**
- **3 cups wheat flour**
- **1 ½ tsp sea salt**
- **2 tbsp olive oil**

1. Mix warm water, yeast, and sugar. Let it sit.
2. Combine flour, salt, olive oil, and yeast mixture. Knead for 6-10 minutes.
3. Coat with olive oil, cover, and let it rise. Heat oven to 500°F.
4. Warm cast iron (10 mins). Divide the dough into 4 balls, cover, and rest for 10 minutes.
5. Roll each ball into a 10-inch circle, dimple with fingers.
6. Bake dough for 5 minutes on a hot surface or in a pan. Transfer baked bread, cover, and repeat with the rest.
7. Serve immediately or store for 3 days at room temp or 1 month in the freezer.

Chicken Gyro

GLUTEN FREE

PREP TIME: 10 MIN **COOK TIME:** 10 MIN **SERVINGS:** 4
Calories: 370, Carbs: 14g, Fat: 16g, Protein: 44g, Fiber: 4g, Sodium: 222mg

- **1 cup yogurt**
- **1 lemon, juiced**
- **2 tbsp olive oil**
- **2 tbsp red wine vinegar**
- **3 garlic cloves, minced**
- **1 tbsp oregano**
- **1 tbsp sweet paprika**
- **1 tsp ground cumin**
- **1 tsp ground coriander**
- **Salt and pepper, to taste**
- **1 ½ lb chicken tenders**
- **1 tbsp olive oil**
- **Pita bread, gluten free**
- **1 tbsp, tzatziki sauce**
- **1 tomato, sliced**
- **1 cucumber, sliced**
- **1 green pepper, sliced**
- **1 onion, sliced**

1. Mix yogurt, lemon juice, olive oil, red wine vinegar, garlic cloves, oregano, paprika, cumin, coriander, season, coat chicken, refrigerate 30 minutes.
2. Heat oil, cook chicken 5 minutes per side until done.
3. Warm pita, add Tzatziki, chicken, veggies (tomato, cucumber, green pepper and onion) wrap, and serve.

Eggplant Pizza

VEGETARIAN

PREP TIME: 10 MIN **COOK TIME:** 20 MIN **SERVINGS:** 6
Calories: 180, Carbs: 9g, Fat: 11g, Protein: 13g, Fiber: 4g, Sodium: 521mg

- **1 eggplant, sliced**
- **Salt, to taste**
- **Olive oil, to taste**
- **2 cups baby spinach**
- **6 oz white mushrooms, sliced**
- **1 cup marinara sauce**
- **10 oz fresh mozzarella**

1. Preheat the oven to 425°F. Season eggplant with salt, let sweat (optional), then wipe off excess moisture.
2. Brush baking sheet with olive oil, arrange eggplant slices, and brush with more oil.
3. Bake for 15-20 minutes, flipping halfway.
4. Cook mushrooms in olive oil for 5 minutes, add spinach, and cook until wilted.
5. Top eggplant with marinara and mozzarella, broil for 1-2 minutes.
6. Add mushroom-spinach mix on top. Serve.

Turkish Steak Wraps

DAIRY FREE

PREP TIME: 10 MIN **COOK TIME:** 15 MIN **SERVINGS:** 6

Calories: 228, Carbs: 1g, Fat: 17g, Protein: 16g, Fiber: 1g, Sodium: 387mg

- 1 small red onion, thinly sliced
- 2 tsp sumac
- Salt, to taste
- 3 Roma tomatoes, finely chopped
- 1 bunch flat-leaf parsley, chopped
- 2 lemons, juiced
- 1 tsp Aleppo pepper (optional)
- 1 ½ lb flank steak
- ¼ cup extra virgin olive oil
- 2 tsp paprika
- 3/4 cup hot water
- 6 sheets homemade lavash (or flour tortillas)

1. Massage onions with sumac and salt.
2. Add tomatoes, parsley, Aleppo pepper, and one lemon juice. Toss.
3. Cook steak in oil for 8 minutes. Add spices and water. Simmer for 5 minutes.
4. Cover steak with lavash. Press for 30 seconds.
5. Add steak and salad to lavash, drizzle with gravy.
6. Roll, squeeze some lemon, and enjoy. Repeat.

Greek New Year's Bread

VEGETARIAN

PREP TIME: 10 MIN **COOK TIME:** 20 MIN **SERVINGS:** 8

Calories: 334, Carbs: 74g, Fat: 3g, Protein: 6g, Fiber: 5g, Sodium: 236mg

- 2 ½ cups granulated sugar
- 2 tsp baking powder
- 1 cup olive oil
- 3 cups Romano cheese, grated
- ½ tsp ground cinnamon
- 2 ½ cup warm water
- 8-10 cups all-purpose flour
- 2 butter sticks, melted
- 1 egg, yolk
- 3 tsp sesame seeds
- ½ cup cinnamon
- 1 cup sugar
- ¼ tsp ground cloves
- ½ tsp allspice
- ½ tsp nutmeg

1. Mix sugar, baking powder, olive oil, 1 cup cheese, and water.
2. Add all-purpose flour gradually, knead for 5 minutes. Let rise.
3. Combine cinnamon, sugar, cloves, allspice, nutmeg. Grease a 10-inch springform pan.
4. Divide dough into 11 balls. Roll each into a 10-inch round.
5. Layer with butter, cinnamon mix, and 2 cups Romano cheese.
6. Repeat until all layers are used. Brush with butter, egg wash, and sesame seeds.
7. Preheat the oven to 350°F. Bake until golden.
8. Cool before slicing.

Flatbread

VEGETARIAN

PREP TIME: 10 MIN **COOK TIME:** 15 MIN **SERVINGS:** 12

Calories: 108, Carbs: 21g, Fat: 1g, Protein: 4g, Fiber: 1g, Sodium: 200mg

- 2 ½ cups bread flour
- 1 tsp instant yeast
- 1 tsp salt
- ⅔ cup warm water
- ⅔ whole milk
- 1 tsp honey

1. Combine flour, yeast, salt, water, milk, and honey.
2. Knead on a floured surface for 3 minutes. Oil bowl, cover dough, and let rise for 45 minutes.
3. Punch down dough, divide into 12 balls. Roll each ball into an 8-inch disc.
4. Cook each disc in a medium skillet for 30-40 seconds per side.
5. Place cooked lavash on a towel to keep warm.
6. Serve warm or store it.

Sesame Bread Rings

VEGETARIAN

PREP TIME: 10 MIN **COOK TIME:** 15 MIN **SERVINGS:** 8

Calories: 506, Carbs: 72g, Fat: 20g, Protein: 14g,
Fiber: 7g, Sodium: 597mg

- ¼ tsp sugar
- 1 tsp dry yeast
- 1 ¾ cups water
- 4 cups flour
- 2 tsp sea salt
- ½ cup grape molasses
- 4 tsp water
- 2 cups sesame seeds

1. Mix sugar, warm water, and yeast. Let foam for 5-8 minutes.
2. Combine flour, salt, and yeast mixture. Stir to form dough. Knead dough, then let rise.
3. Preheat to 400°F. Line 2 baking sheets. Mix molasses and water, pour sesame seeds on a plate.
4. Divide dough into 8, roll into 24-inch ropes. Twist into circles.
5. Dip rings in molasses mixture, coat in sesame seeds.
6. Let it rest for 15 minutes. Bake until golden. Cool on a wire rack.

Greek Pizza

VEGETARIAN

PREP TIME: 05 MIN **COOK TIME:** 25 MIN **SERVINGS:** 8

Calories: 348, Carbs: 33g, Fat: 22g, Protein: 5g, Fiber: 3g, Sodium: 428mg

- 1 tsp instant yeast
- 1 tsp castor sugar
- 1 ½ cups water
- 2 ½ cups flour
- ¼ cup olive oil
- 1 tsp salt
- 2 tomatoes, sliced
- 1 onion, sliced
- 1 tbsp oregano
- ½ cup olive oil
- ½ cup kalamata olives
- ¾ cup feta cheese

1. Combine yeast, sugar, and water. Add flour, ¼ cup olive oil, salt; mix into dough.
2. Coat pan with olive oil, press dough to edges.
3. Cover and let rise for 30 mins. Mix tomatoes, onion, oregano, ½ cup olive oil, kalamata olives and salt.
4. Set the oven to 400°F. Stretch dough, add feta, tomato mix.
5. Bake until golden. Slice and enjoy.

Phyllo-Wrapped Greek Baked Feta with Honey

VEGETARIAN

PREP TIME: 05 MIN **COOK TIME:** 20 MIN **SERVINGS:** 6

Calories: 74, Carbs: 15g, Fat: 7g, Protein: 1g, Fiber: 1g, Sodium: 16mg

- 2 blocks feta, 3 oz
- 2 sheets phyllo dough, thawed
- ¼ cup honey
- 2 tbsp sesame seeds
- 1 tbsp thyme, for garnish

1. Preheat the oven to 350°F. Brush phyllo with olive oil.
2. Wrap feta in phyllo, folding edges, brush with oil.
3. Bake for 20 minutes, turning if needed.
4. Serve with honey, sesame seeds, and thyme.

Persian Flatbread

VEGETARIAN

PREP TIME: 10 MIN **COOK TIME:** 20 MIN **SERVINGS:** 10

Calories: 204, Carbs: 38g, Fat: 3g, Protein: 7g,
Fiber: 2g, Sodium: 489mg

- 1 packet dry yeast
- 1 ⅓ cups tepid water
- 1 tsp sugar
- 4 cups purpose flour
- 1 tsp olive oil
- 2 tsp salt
- 1 tbsp flour
- ½ tsp baking powder
- ⅓ cup water
- 1 tsp olive oil
- Sesame seeds, to garnish

1. Mix tepid water, yeast, and sugar. Let sit for 15 minutes.
2. Combine flour, 1 tsp oil, salt, and yeast mixture. Stir into dough. Knead dough for 5-10 minutes until smooth.
3. Let rise for 1 hour. Mix ⅓ cup water, 1 tbsp flour, baking powder, and 1 tsp oil into a paste. Set it aside.
4. Punch down and divide the dough in half.
5. Roll dough into 11x8 inches, score, and press for ridges.
6. Let rise for 30 minutes.
7. Preheat the oven to 425°F. Brush with glaze, top with seeds, bake.

CHAPTER 13
DESSERTS

Let's satisfy your sweet tooth Mediterranean-style! In this chapter, we'll dive into delicious, simple desserts that bring the perfect balance of flavors and textures.

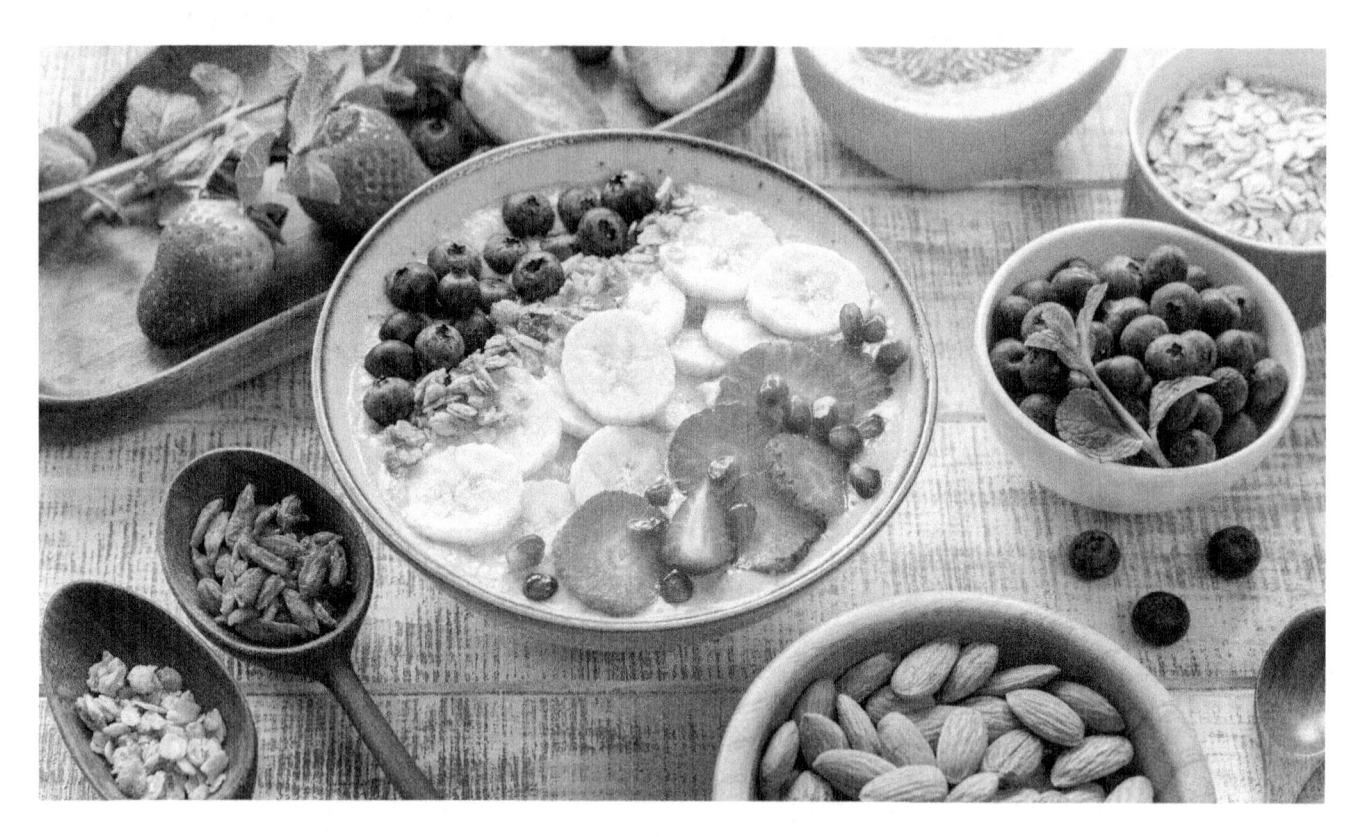

TIPS

- For natural sweetness, drizzle honey over your desserts—it's a Mediterranean staple that adds richness and flavor.

- Mediterranean desserts often highlight fresh, seasonal fruit. Think figs, oranges, and berries for a light, refreshing touch.

- Greek yogurt is a great way to balance sweetness in desserts—serve it alongside pastries or drizzle it on top of cakes.

French Pear Tart

VEGETARIAN

PREP TIME: 10 MIN **COOK TIME:** 30 MIN **SERVINGS:** 12
Calories: 431, Carbs: 58g, Fat: 22g, Protein: 3g, Fiber: 5g, Sodium: 189mg

- 1 ½ cups all-purpose flour
- 5 tbsp sugar
- ½ tsp salt
- 12 tbsp unsalted butter
- 8 pears, washed
- 3 tbsp unsalted butter
- 1 tbsp water
- ¾ cup fig preserves
- ¼ tsp salt

1. Preheat oven to 350°F. Position one rack in the middle and another at the top.
2. Mix flour, sugar, ½ tsp salt, and melted butter to form dough. Press into a 9-inch tart pan.
3. Bake until golden. Let cool.
4. Microwave fig preserves for 40 seconds and strain to remove chunks.
5. Slice 5 pears, cook in 1 tbsp butter with 1 tbsp water for 3 minutes. Set it aside.
6. Slice the remaining 3 pears. In the same pan, cook with butter, fig chunks, and ¼ tsp salt for 10 minutes, then mash.
7. Spread pear-fig puree over cooled crust.
8. Arrange pear slices on top in circles and bake.
9. Brush with fig liquid and broil briefly until caramelized.
10. Cool for 1 ½ hours, then remove from pan.
11. Slice it into 8 pieces and serve. Enjoy!

Pignoli Cookies

VEGETARIAN

PREP TIME: 15 MIN **COOK TIME:** 15 MIN **SERVINGS:** 12
Calories: 185, Carbs: 18g, Fat: 13g, Protein: 4g, Fiber: 1g, Sodium: 55mg

- 7 oz almond paste
- ½ cup granulated sugar
- 1 egg, white
- ¼ tsp salt
- 1 cup pine nuts

1. Preheat the oven to 350°F. Line a baking sheet with parchment.
2. Blend almond paste, sugar, egg white, and salt in a food processor until smooth.
3. Roll into 12 balls. Chill if needed. Roll balls in pine nuts, pressing to stick. Place on sheet, 2 inches apart.
4. Bake until golden. Let cool completely.

Mango Strawberry Smoothie with Greek Yogurt

VEGETARIAN, GLUTEN FREE

PREP TIME: 10 MIN **COOK TIME:** 00 MIN **SERVINGS:** 4
Calories: 171, Carbs: 35g, Fat: 2g, Protein: 7g, Fiber: 3g, Sodium: 31mg

- ½ cup frozen strawberries
- ¼ tsp turmeric
- ½ cup frozen mango
- 1 banana
- ¼ tsp ginger
- ½ cup Greek yogurt
- 1 tbsp honey
- ¼ cup almond milk

1. Add all the ingredients in a food processor and blend.

Pear Cake

VEGETARIAN

PREP TIME: 10 MIN **COOK TIME:** 25 MIN **SERVINGS:** 10
Calories: 308, Carbs: 46g, Fat: 12g, Protein: 5g, Fiber: 2g, Sodium: 218mg

- 2 cups flour
- 2 tsp baking powder
- ½ tsp salt
- 2 eggs
- 1 cup granulated sugar
- 1 lemon, zested
- 1 orange, zested
- ½ cup olive oil
- ½ cup yogurt
- 1 tsp vanilla extract
- 2 large pears, cut into wedges
- Powdered sugar, for dusting

1. Preheat the oven to 350°F. Grease a 9-inch springform pan.
2. Whisk flour, baking powder, and salt and put aside. Beat eggs, sugar, and zest until pale and doubled, about 3 minutes.
3. Slowly add olive oil while beating. Stir in yogurt and vanilla.
4. Fold in dry ingredients until combined.
5. Pour batter into pan, top with pear wedges. Bake in the oven. Cool for 30 minutes.
6. Release from pan, dust with powdered sugar, slice, and serve.

Traditional Greek Orange Cake

VEGETARIAN
PREP TIME: 05 MIN **COOK TIME:** 25 MIN **SERVINGS:** 6
Calories: 495, Carbs: 70g, Fat: 23g, Protein: 6g, Fiber: 1g, Sodium: 376mg

- ½ cup orange juice
- 1 ½ cups water
- 1 cup honey
- ½ cup granulated sugar or coconut sugar
- 1 lb phyllo dough
- 5 large eggs
- ¾ cup granulated sugar
- 1 tbsp baking powder
- 1 cup olive oil
- 1 cup yogurt
- 1 ¼ cups orange juice and zested
- 1 tsp vanilla extract
- ¼ tsp salt

1. Preheat the oven to 350°F. Grease a 9x14-inch pan.
2. Use a sharp knife to peel off one orange, leaving the white pith behind.
3. Boil orange peel, ½ cup of orange juice, water, honey, and sugar for 5 minutes. Cool.
4. Tear phyllo into strips, bake.
5. Beat eggs and sugar. Add baking powder, oil, yogurt, zest, 1 ¼ juice, vanilla, and salt.
6. Fold in toasted phyllo. Pour into the pan, bake until golden.
7. Pour syrup over cake and let sit for 30 minutes. Slice it into 12 pieces.

Chocolate Hazelnut Cookies

VEGETARIAN
PREP TIME: 10 MIN **COOK TIME:** 18 MIN **SERVINGS:** 28
Calories: 50, Carbs: 5g, Fat: 4g, Protein: 1g, Fiber: 1g, Sodium: 13mg

- 1 cup raw hazelnuts, unsalted
- ¾ cup granulated coconut sugar
- 1 cup almond flour
- ¼ tsp salt
- ¼ cup coconut oil or olive oil
- 1 tsp vanilla extract
- 1 tsp lemon zest
- 4 oz dark chocolate

1. Preheat oven to 350°F, line baking sheets using parchment paper.
2. Toast hazelnuts for 10 minutes, rub off skins.
3. Process hazelnuts with sugar, then add flour and salt, blend.
4. Add coconut oil, vanilla, lemon zest, and pulse until dough forms.
5. Shape into logs, cut into 24 pieces, roll into balls, and place on sheets.
6. Bake until golden. Let cool.
7. Melt chocolate in 30-second intervals, stir smoothly.
8. Spread ½ tsp chocolate on one cookie, sandwich with another.

Lemon Sorbet

VEGETARIAN, GLUTEN FREE, DAIRY FREE
PREP TIME: 05 MIN **COOK TIME:** 20 MIN
SERVINGS: 20
Calories: 164, Carbs: 9g, Fat: 11g, Protein: 7g, Fiber: 1g, Sodium: 461mg

- ⅔ cup lemon juice with its peel
- ¾ cup coconut sugar
- Mint leaves, for garnish

1. Place a stainless-steel mixing bowl in the freezer.
2. Peel lemon zest, avoiding pith. Set lemons aside.
3. Heat sugar, lemon zest, and 1 cup water until sugar dissolves. Cool for 45 minutes, then remove zest.
4. Strain and juice lemons, refrigerate.
5. Blend syrup and lemon juice until frothy.
6. Pour into chilled bowl and freeze.
7. Spoon into glasses, garnish with mint, and enjoy!

Poached Apricots with Ricotta

VEGETARIAN, GLUTEN FREE
PREP TIME: 10 MIN **COOK TIME:** 20 MIN **SERVINGS:** 12
Calories: 127, Carbs: 26g, Fat: 3g, Protein: 3g, Fiber: 2g, Sodium: 12mg

- ⅔ cup granulated sugar or coconut sugar
- 2 cups hot water
- 1 tbsp lemon juice
- 9 oz dried apricots
- 4 ½ oz whole milk ricotta
- 2 tbsp unsalted pistachios

1. Boil sugar and water, then simmer on medium-low.
2. Add lemon juice and apricots.
3. Simmer, then cool. Cut slits in apricots. Fill cooled apricots with ricotta.
4. Drizzle with syrup and top with pistachios.

Candied Almonds

VEGETARIAN, GLUTEN FREE, DAIRY FREE
PREP TIME: 05 MIN **COOK TIME:** 25 MIN **SERVINGS:** 6
Calories: 280, Carbs: 32g, Fat: 16g, Protein: 7g, Fiber: 4g, Sodium: 74mg

- 1 ¾ cups raw almonds
- 1 cup sugar
- ½ cup water
- 1 tsp vanilla extract
- ¼ tsp salt
- 1 tsp ground cinnamon

1. Line a baking sheet with parchment paper.
2. Combine almonds, sugar, water, vanilla, salt, and cinnamon in a pan.
3. Bring to a boil for 3-5 minutes. Reduce heat and simmer, stirring until syrup thickens and crystallizes.
4. Increase heat, stir until sugar melts and coats almonds. Cook for 4-5 minutes.
5. Transfer almonds to the sheet, separate them, and cool completely.

Tiramisu

VEGETARIAN
PREP TIME: 05 MIN **COOK TIME:** 20 MIN **SERVINGS:** 8
Calories: 434, Carbs: 28g, Fat: 30g, Protein: 11g, Fiber: 1g, Sodium: 112mg

- 4 large eggs
- 2 cups mascarpone cheese
- ¼ cups granulated sugar
- ½ cup strong coffee
- 24 ladyfinger cookies
- Cocoa powder, for dusting

1. Beat egg whites until stiff peaks form. Beat egg yolks and sugar until pale and thick.
2. Add mascarpone to the yolk mixture, then fold in egg whites.
3. Dip half the ladyfingers in coffee, arrange in a pan.
4. Spread half the mascarpone mixture over ladyfingers, then add another layer of dipped ladyfingers and remaining mascarpone.
5. Refrigerate for 6 hours or overnight.
6. Dust with cocoa powder and serve.

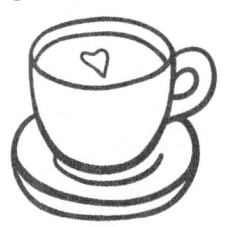

Fruit Salad with Citrus Honey Dressing

VEGETARIAN, GLUTEN FREE
PREP TIME: 10 MIN **COOK TIME:** 05 MIN **SERVINGS:** 4
Calories: 135, Carbs: 25g, Fat: 4g, Protein: 2g, Fiber: 5g, Sodium: 2.2mg

- 3 lemons, juiced
- 3 tbsp honey
- ½ tsp rose water
- 2 cups strawberries, sliced
- 1 cup cherries, pitted and halved
- ½ cup raspberries
- 1 cup blackberries
- ¼ cup pomegranate seeds
- ⅓ cup walnuts, chopped
- 2 tbsp mint leaves

1. Heat lemon juice and honey in a saucepan until warm, about 2 minutes. Remove from heat, stir in rosewater (optional), and set aside to cool.
2. Combine strawberries, cherries, blackberries, raspberries, and pomegranate seeds in a bowl. Toss with dressing.
3. Add walnuts and mint, toss again, and serve.

Greek Rice Pudding

VEGETARIAN
PREP TIME: 05 MIN **COOK TIME:** 25 MIN **SERVINGS:** 4
Calories: 282, Carbs: 41g, Fat: 9g, Protein: 11g, Fiber: 2g, Sodium: 100mg

- 4 ¼ cups whole milk
- ½ cup Arborio rice
- 1 cinnamon stick
- 1 tsp vanilla extract
- 2-inch, lemon rind
- Zest of ¼ orange
- 1 tbsp cornstarch
- 2 tbsp sugar
- Ground cinnamon, for garnish

1. In a saucepan, combine milk, rice, cinnamon stick, lemon peel, and orange zest.
2. Heat to a simmer over medium-low, whisking for 3 minutes.
3. Simmer while stirring occasionally, until rice is soft, and the mixture thickens.
4. Mix cornstarch with water, stir into the mixture, and cook until thickened. Remove from heat.
5. Remove cinnamon stick and lemon peel. Add vanilla and sugar to taste.
6. Pour into bowls, top with cinnamon, and serve warm, at room temperature, or chilled.

Rose Water Milk Pudding

VEGETARIAN, GLUTEN FREE
PREP TIME: 15 MIN **COOK TIME:** 10 MIN **SERVINGS:** 8
Calories: 192, Carbs: 34g, Fat: 5g, Protein: 5g, Fiber: 2g, Sodium: 48mg

- 4 cups whole milk
- ½ cup granulated coconut sugar
- ½ cup cornstarch
- 1 tsp rosewater
- 2 tbsp unsalted shelled pistachios
- 1 lb strawberries
- 2 tbsp coconut sugar
- ½ tsp rosewater

1. Whisk milk, sugar, and cornstarch in a saucepan.
2. Heat until it boils, then simmer and thicken for 10 minutes.
3. Stir in rose water and remove from heat. Pour into cups and refrigerate for 2-3 hours.
4. Mix strawberries, sugar, and rosewater.
5. Let sit for 30 minutes to 2 hours. Refrigerate until ready.
6. Top pudding with strawberries and crushed pistachios. Serve cold.

Italian Carrot Cake

VEGETARIAN
PREP TIME: 15 MIN **COOK TIME:** 20 MIN **SERVINGS:** 10
Calories: 280, Carbs: 35g, Fat: 14g, Protein: 9g, Fiber: 4g, Sodium: 229mg

- 2 cups, almond flour
- ⅔ cups all-purpose flour
- 1 tbsp baking powder
- 1 cup organic cane sugar
- 1 orange, zested
- 5 eggs, separated
- 3 large carrots
- 1 tsp almond extract
- ¼ tsp salt
- ¼ cup honey

1. Set to 350°F. Grease and line a 9-inch cake pan.
2. Spread almond flour on a baking sheet. Toast stirring halfway. Cool completely.
3. Sift together flour, baking powder, and toasted almond flour.
4. Rub orange zest into sugar. Add egg yolks and whisk until pale and fluffy.
5. Mix in sifted flour, shredded carrots, and almond extract.
6. Beat egg whites with salt until stiff peaks form. Gently fold whipped egg whites into batter.
7. Pour into the prepared pan. Bake, rotating halfway, until golden.
8. Let the cake cool completely, then remove from the pan.
9. Dust with powdered sugar, drizzle with honey, and top with Greek yogurt.

Burbura

DAIRY FREE, VEGETARIAN
PREP TIME: 05 MIN **COOK TIME:** 25 MIN **SERVINGS:** 6
Calories: 213, Carbs: 51g, Fat: 0.6g, Protein: 4.1g, Fiber: 7g, Sodium: 9.9mg

- 1 cup pearled barley
- 4 cups water
- 1 tsp ground cinnamon
- 4 tbsp brown sugar
- 1 tsp anise seeds
- ½ tsp fennel seeds
- ½ cup chopped apricots, dried
- ½ cup raisins, dried
- Pomegranate seeds, for garnish

1. Combine barley and water in a saucepan. Bring to a boil, then simmer, stirring occasionally.
2. Add cinnamon, sugar, anise seeds, fennel seeds, and dried fruit.
3. Cook until the barley is tender.
4. Serve topped with nuts, dried fruit, and pomegranate seeds. Refrigerate leftovers.

Crema Catalana

VEGETARIAN, GLUTEN FREE
PREP TIME: 10 MIN **COOK TIME:** 10 MIN **SERVINGS:** 6
Calories: 290, Carbs: 39g, Fat: 12g, Protein: 10g, Fiber: 0.7g, Sodium: 268mg

- ¾ cups granulated sugar
- 3 tbsp cornstarch
- ½ tsp salt
- 8 eggs, yolks
- 4 cups whole milk
- 1 strip lemon zest
- 1 strip orange zest
- 1 cinnamon stick

1. For preparation: Set a sieve over a bowl. Arrange six 6-ounce ramekins.
2. Mix sugar, cornstarch, salt, and egg yolks until smooth.
3. Simmer milk, lemon zest, orange zest, and

cinnamon in a pan.
4. Remove from heat. Slowly whisk hot milk into egg mixture.
5. Return to pan and cook over medium-low, whisking until thickened and simmering.
6. Strain custard, pour into ramekins, cover, and chill for 4 hours or overnight.
7. Sprinkle sugar on top and use a kitchen torch to caramelize.
8. Serve immediately.

Berry Compote

VEGETARIAN, DAIRY FREE, GLUTEN FREE
PREP TIME: 05 MIN **COOK TIME:** 25 MIN
SERVINGS: 3 ½ CUPS
Calories: 11, Carbs: 3g, Fat: 0,1g, Protein: 0.2g, Fiber: 0.7g, Sodium: 0.2mg

- 12 oz fresh strawberries
- 12 oz fresh blueberries
- 12 oz fresh raspberries
- 3 tbsp raw cane sugar
- Juice of 1 lime

1. Combine fruits, sugar, and lime juice in a saucepan.
2. Boil over medium-high heat for 5 minutes. Reduce heat to low and let it simmer.
3. Mash if desired, adjust sweetness if needed.
4. Cool for 15-30 minutes before serving.

Italian Chocolate Cake

VEGETARIAN
PREP TIME: 05 MIN **COOK TIME:** 25 MIN **SERVINGS:** 8
Calories: 450, Carbs: 31g, Fat: 34g, Protein: 9g, Fiber: 3g, Sodium: 121mg

- 5 oz dark chocolate
- 11 tbsp unsalted butter
- ⅔ cup granulated sugar
- ¼ tsp salt
- 3 eggs
- ¾ cup almond flour

1. Preheat the oven to 350°F. Grease and line an 8–10-inch cake pans. Melt chocolate.
2. Beat butter, sugar, and salt until smooth.
3. Add eggs and almond flour, mix. Stir in melted chocolate.
4. Pour batter into the pan and bake until the toothpick comes out clean.
5. Cool completely, remove from pan, dust with powdered sugar, and serve after 30 minutes.

Tahini Banana Date Shake

VEGETARIAN, GLUTEN FREE, DAIRY FREE
PREP TIME: 10 MIN **COOK TIME:** 00 MIN **SERVINGS:** 2
Calories: 299, Carbs: 47g, Fat: 12g, Protein: 5g, Fiber: 0g, Sodium: 102mg

- 2 frozen bananas, sliced
- 4 pitted medjool dates
- ¼ cup tahini
- ¼ cup crushed ice
- 1 ½ cups unsweetened almond milk
- Ground cinnamon, a pinch

1. Add all the ingredients to a blender.
2. Blend until a smooth consistency is achieved.

Fig Pastry

VEGETARIAN, GLUTEN FREE
PREP TIME: 10 MIN **COOK TIME:** 20 MIN **SERVINGS:** 4
Calories: 240, Carbs: 22g, Fat: 15g, Protein: 7g, Fiber: 2g, Sodium: 3mg

- 1 sheet puff pastry
- 8 oz fresh black mission figs
- 4-5 oz goat cheese
- ¼ cup walnuts
- 2 tbsp good fig jam
- 1 tbsp butter
- ⅓ cup mint leaves

1. Preheat the oven to 375°F.
2. Cut the puff pastry into 4 rectangles and place on a baking sheet. Spread goat cheese, then add jam, figs, and walnuts.
3. Brush with melted butter and fold pastry edges. Bake until golden.
4. Garnish with mint and walnuts.

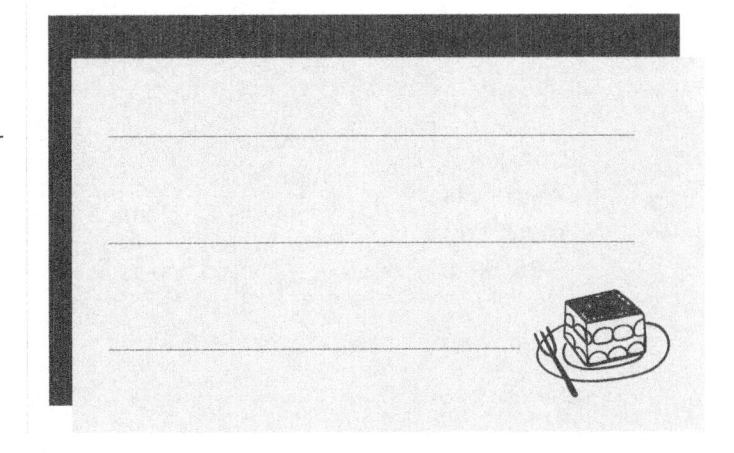

MEAL PLAN 1-7 DAYS

The Mediterranean diet is all about enjoying fresh, flavorful foods while keeping things simple and healthy. To help you get started, we've included a meal plan and a shopping list to make things easy. With these, you'll spend less time planning and more time enjoying delicious, wholesome meals.

Day	Breakfast	Snack	Lunch	Snack	Dinner	Calories
1	Buckwheat Pancakes 572kcal	Greek Yogurt with Honey, Walnuts, and Spiced Raisin Syrup 195kcal	Turkish-Style Marinated Salmon 386kcal	Steamed Artichokes With Avocado Tahini Dressing 220kcal	Saffron Chicken 586kcal	1959
2	Turkish Poached Eggs 343kcal	Greek Rice Pudding 282kcal	Chicken Pesto Pasta 445kcal	Eggplant Pizza 370kcal	Egyptian Fried Fish Sandwich 308kcal	1748
3	Mediterranean Scramble With Lemon Zest And Spinach 175kcal	Mango Strawberry Smoothie with Greek Yogurt 171kcal	Lentils and Rice with Caramelized Onions 448kcal	Italian Carrot Cake 280kcal	Tuna Pasta with Peas 538kcal	1612
4	Lemon Herb Millet Porridge Garlic-Infused Oil 190kcal	Tahini Banana Date Shake 299kcal	Cod And Potato Chowder 240kcal	Garlic Dijon Chicken 198kcal	Spanish Rice and Beans 487kcal	1414
5	Lebanese Potatoes and Eggs 265kcal	Majorcan Vegetable Flatbread 180kcal	Black Olive Tapenade With Pasta 537kcal	Mediterranean Wrap 210kcal	Apricot Chicken 356kcal	1548
6	Pastilla (Skillet Chicken Pie) 382kcal	Crema Catalana 290kcal	Kleftiko (Greek Lamb Cooked in Parchment) 328kcal	Pignoli Cookies 185kcal	Lemony Shrimp Risotto 523kcal	1708
7	Pomegranate & Walnut Greek Yogurt Parfait 250kcal	Coconut Turmeric Vegetable Stew 220kcal	Chicken in Tomato Sauce 228kcal	Zucchini Noodles With Almond Pesto And Roasted Vegetables 180kcal	Albondigas (Spanish Meatballs) 401kcal	1279

MEAL PLAN 8-14 DAYS

Day	Breakfast	Snack	Lunch	Snack	Dinner	Calories
8	Tunisian Brik au Thon **335kcal**	Sesame Bread Rings **506kcal**	Stifado (Greek Beef Stew) **475kcal**	Fruit Salad with Citrus Honey Dressing **135kcal**	Greek Chicken Marinade **247kcal**	1698
9	Risotto Radicchio and Gorgonzola **640kcal**	Fig Pastry **240kcal**	Roast Turkey Breast **255kcal**	Candied Almonds **280kcal**	Vegetarian Pizza **301kcal**	1716
10	Orange And Pistachio Breakfast Bowl With Almond Flakes And Mint **195kcal**	Tiramisu **434kcal**	Spaghetti with Garlicky Sautéed Shrimp **462kcal**	Rose Water Milk Pudding **192kcal**	Spiced Lamb And Vegetable Soup **190kcal**	1473
11	Mediterranean Bowl with Quinoa, Hummus, and Harissa **325kcal**	French Pear Tart **431kcal**	Creamy Salmon Soup **250kcal**	Mussels with Chorizo **260kcal**	Chicken Saltimbocca **360kcal**	1626
12	Mediterranean Avocado And Nut Bowl With Lemon-Oregano Drizzle **270kcal**	Greek Meatloaf Wrapped in Grape Leaves **195kcal**	Linguine with Clams **424kcal**	Smashed Chickpea Toast **126kcal**	Mediterranean Fish Fillet **469kcal**	1484
13	Spanakopita Egg Muffins + Tahini Banana Date Shake **438kcal**	Burbura **213kcal**	Herb Beef Soup **328kcal**	Lemon Sorbet **164kcal**	Mediterranean Salmon kabobs **479kcal**	1622
14	Citrus Bliss Yogurt Parfait **210kcal**	Sun-Dried Tomato Chickpea Pancakes With Herbed Toppings **230kcal**	Steamed Mussels in Garlic White Wine Broth **332kcal**	Spiced Sweet Potato & Date Delight **240kcal**	Baked Tomato Chicken Thighs with Couscous **627kcal**	1639

MEAL PLAN 15-22 DAY

Day	Breakfast	Snack	Lunch	Snack	Dinner	Calories
15	Sun-Kissed Chickpea And Avocado Breakfast Bowl 250kcal	Soft Scrambled Eggs With Chives 206kcal	Sheet Pan Za'atar Chicken With Veggies 465kcal	Greek New Year's Bread 334kcal	Mediterranean Oven Roasted Spanish Mackerel 239kcal	1494
16	Smoky Sweet Potato Breakfast Hash 230kcal	Pistachio Chia Banana Bowl 230kcal	Chicken Gyro 370kcal	Greek Pizza 348kcal	Italian Steak With Arugula And Parmesan 429kcal	1607
17	Cinnamon Figs & Seeds Porridge 280kcal	Mediterranean-Spiced Tofu Scramble With Bell Peppers And Tomato 150kcal	Pan Seared Lamb Chops 506kcal	Quinoa Olive Crisp Bites 130kcal	Mediterranean-Style Whole Roasted Red Snapper 344kcal	1410
18	Sunrise Quinoa Delight 270kcal	Tahini Banana Date Shake 299kcal	Smoky Chicken And Butternut Squash Soup + Tunisian Salad 458kcal	Cranberry Apple Freekeh Stuffing 230kcal	Joojeh Kabob + Greek Lemon Rice 396kcal	1653
19	Savory Tomato-Basil Omelet+ Mango Strawberry Smoothie With Greek Yogurt 471kcal	Grilled Steak Salad With Balsamic Vinaigrette 265kcal	Hearty Turkey Meatball And Kale Soup + Roasted Bell Peppers With Olive Tapenade 340kcal	Chocolate Hazelnut Cookies 50kcal	Apricot Chicken 356kcal	1482
20	Italina Eggs In Purgatory 208kcal	Caramelized Rutabaga With Miso Glaze 190kcal	Sausage And Lentils With Fennel 327kcal	Palestinian Flatbread 536kcal	Ocean Kissed Tomato Soup With Sea Bass 130kcal	1391
21	Pomegranate & Walnut Greek Yogurt Parfait 250kcal	Roasted Cauliflower And Chickpea Salad With Lemon-Tahini Dressing 280kcal	Mussels Marinara With Fennel (Greece) 228kcal	Spinach & Pine Nut Puff Rolls 160kcal	Albondigas (Spanish Meatballs) 401kcal	1319
22	Cinnamon Figs & Seeds Porridge 280kcal	Pistachio Chia Banana Bowl 230kcal	Pan Seared Lamb Chops 506kcal	Cranberry Apple Freekeh Stuffing 230kcal	Mediterranean Oven Roasted Spanish Mackerel 239kcal	1485

MEAL PLAN 23-30 DAY

Day	Breakfast	Snack	Lunch	Snack	Dinner	Calories
23	Buckwheat Pancakes **572kcal**	Mango Strawberry Smoothie with Greek Yogurt **171kcal**	Cod And Potato Chowder **240kcal**	Shrimp Fra Diavolo **194kcal**	Chicken Pesto Pasta **445kcal**	1622
24	Lemon Herb Millet Porridge Garlic-Infused Oil **190kcal**	Greek Rice Pudding **282kcal**	Saffron Chicken **586kcal**	Italian Carrot Cake **280kcal**	Egyptian Fried Fish Sandwich **308kcal**	1646
25	Lebanese Potatoes and Eggs **265kcal**	Greek Yogurt with Honey, Walnuts, and Spiced Raisin Syrup **195kcal**	Chicken Gyro **370kcal**	Eggplant Pizza **370kcal**	Tuna Pasta with Peas **538kcal**	1738
26	Garbanzo Bean Pilaf **276kcal**	Italian Chocolate Cake **450kcal**	Turkish-Style Marinated Salmon **386kcal**	Garlic Dijon Chicken **198kcal**	Spanish Rice and Beans **487kcal**	1797
27	Mediterranean Scramble With Lemon Zest And Spinach **175kcal**	Crema Catalana **290kcal**	Black Olive Tapenade With Pasta **537kcal**	Tahini Banana Date Shake **299kcal**	Apricot Chicken **356kcal**	1657
28	Pastilla (Skillet Chicken Pie) **382kcal**	Fig Pastry **240kcal**	Kleftiko (Greek Lamb Cooked in Parchment) **328kcal**	Easy Mediterranean Sautéed Scallops **234kcal**	Tunisian Chickpea Stew **196kcal**	1380
29	White Bean Shakshuka **115kcal**	Coconut Turmeric Vegetable Stew **220kcal**	Chicken in Tomato Sauce **228kcal**	Pear Cake **308kcal**	Black Bean Avocado Quinoa Bowl **500kcal**	1371
30	Lebanese Potatoes and Eggs **265kcal**	Majorcan Vegetable Flatbread **180kcal**	Black Olive Tapenade With Pasta **537kcal**	Mussels with Chorizo **260kcal**	Chicken Saltimbocca **360kcal**	1602

For detailed shopping lists, please download via https://heartbookspress.com/SuperEasyMediterranean-FreeBonuses

CONVERSIONS AND EQUIVALENTS

Precision is the secret ingredient to cooking success. Using accurate measurements not only ensures that your dishes turn out delicious every time but also keeps your anti-inflammatory meals consistent and balanced. This Cooking Conversion Chart is here to guide you through the essentials, making your time in the kitchen smooth and enjoyable.

Volume Conversions
- 1 cup = 16 tablespoons
- 1 tablespoon = 3 teaspoons
- 1 fluid ounce = 2 tablespoons = 6 teaspoons
- 1 pint = 2 cups = 16 fluid ounces
- 1 quart = 4 cups = 32 fluid ounces
- 1 gallon = 4 quarts = 16 cups = 128 fluid ounces

Weight Conversions
- 1 ounce = 28 grams
- 1 pound = 16 ounces = 454 grams
- 1 kilogram = 1000 grams = 2.2 pounds

Temperature Equivalents
Converting between temperature scales is a breeze with these simple formulas:
- To convert °F to °C: (°F - 32) × 5/9
- To convert °C to °F: (°C × 9/5) + 32

For example, 350°F converts to approximately 176.67°C. Having these conversions at your fingertips ensures your recipes turn out perfectly, no matter the temperature settings.

Common Ingredient Equivalents
Accurate ingredient measurements can make all the difference in achieving the perfect dish. Here are some useful conversions for everyday ingredients:
- 1 medium banana ≈ 1/2 cup mashed banana
- 1 large egg = 2 small eggs or 3 medium eggs
- 1 cup grated cheese = 4 ounces
- 1 cup breadcrumbs = 4 slices of bread
- 1 cup chopped nuts = 4.5 ounces
- 1 cup cooked rice = 1/2 cup uncooked rice
- 1 cup cooked pasta = 2 ounces uncooked pasta
- 1 stick of butter = 1/2 cup = 8 tablespoons = 4 ounce

CONCLUSION

Thank you for choosing to embrace a healthier, happier lifestyle with the Mediterranean way of eating. Whether you're just starting or already enjoying its vibrant flavors, every small change and bite is a step toward a better you.

Remember, this isn't about perfection—it's about progress. The Mediterranean diet is about living fully, enjoying food, and nourishing your body with simple, delicious ingredients.

I've created this cookbook to make healthy eating simple, quick, and affordable, perfect for even the busiest days. Change isn't always easy, especially in a busy world and healthy eating shouldn't add to that stress.

What excites me most about the Mediterranean lifestyle is that it's not just about food—it's about creating memories, savoring meals, and reconnecting with the joy of cooking.

This book is more than just recipes; it's an invitation to rethink how we approach food and life.

Make room for the foods you love, and remember, every positive change counts.

I hope this book serves as a go-to guide for inspiration, even on your busiest days. Healthy eating doesn't have to be complicated—enjoy the journey, relish the flavors, and celebrate every step.

Thank you for joining me on this Mediterranean adventure. May your meals nourish your body and soul, and may your life be filled with health, happiness, and joy!

With deepest appreciation,

Elena Florenz

THANK YOU

Thank you so much for purchasing my cookbook.

You could have picked from dozens of other cookbooks but you took a chance and chose this one. I hope you've found inspiration in *The Super Easy & Practical Mediterranean Diet Cookbook for Beginners: Optimize Your Health with Budget Friendly, Quick & Tasty 30-Minute, 5-ingredient Healthy Recipes + A 30-Day Meal Plan* to get you started on your journey to great health and happiness.

So *THANK YOU* for getting this book.

Before you go, I wanted to ask you for one small favor. **Could you please consider posting a review on the platform? Posting a review is the best and easiest way to support the work of independent authors like me.**

Your review will help me keep writing the kind of cookbooks that will help you get the results you want. It would mean a lot to me to hear from you.

Leave a review on Amazon US

Leave a review on Amazon UK

Leave a review on Amazon CA

REFERENCES

American Heart Association. (2020). *The Mediterranean diet: A heart-healthy eating plan.* American Heart Association. https://www.heart.org/en/healthy-living/healthy-eating/eat-smart/nutrition-basics/mediterranean-diet

Gibney, M. J., & L. J. L. (2021). *The Mediterranean diet and its health benefits.* Nutrition Reviews, 79(5), 345-359. https://doi.org/10.1093/nutrit/nuab025

Hawkes, C. (2021). *The role of shared meals in promoting emotional well-being and reducing stress.* Journal of Social and Clinical Psychology, 40(2), 110-118. https://doi.org/10.1521/jscp.2021.40.2.110

López-Miranda, J., & Pérez-Martínez, P. (2022). *The Mediterranean diet and cardiovascular disease prevention: A comprehensive review.* Nutrients, 14(3), 597. https://doi.org/10.3390/nu14030597

Ramos, S. B., & Moreira, L. (2021). *Shared meals as a cornerstone of family well-being and nutrition.* Journal of Family Studies, 32(1), 62-78. https://doi.org/10.1080/13229400.2021.1888347

Schwarz, L. M., & Thompson, J. R. (2023). *Health benefits of Mediterranean-style diets: Evidence and practice.* Health & Wellness, 21(4), 34-46. https://www.healthandwellnessjournal.com/mediterranean-diets

Wahlqvist, M. L., & Tricon, S. (2022). *The science of the Mediterranean diet and its impact on longevity and cognitive health.* Aging and Nutrition, 15(4), 231-239. https://doi.org/10.1007/agingnutrition2022.08.04

Printed in Great Britain
by Amazon